BASIC CONCEPTS IN PHARMACOLOGY

A STUDENT'S SURVIVAL GUIDE

JANET L. STRINGER, M.D., Ph.D.
Department of Pharmacology and Division of Neuroscience
Baylor College of Medicine
Houston, Texas

The McGraw-Hill Companies
Health Professions Division

New York   St. Louis   San Francisco
Auckland   Bogota   Caracus   Lisbon   London   Madrid
Mexico City   Milan   Montreal   New Delhi   Paris   San Juan
Singapore   Sydney   Tokyo   Toronto

McGraw-Hill

*A Division of The **McGraw·Hill** Companies*

BASIC CONCEPTS IN PHARMACOLOGY:
A STUDENT'S SURVIVAL GUIDE

4 5 6 7 8 9 0 DOC DOC 9

ISBN 0-07-063165-4

This book was set in Times Roman by Huron Valley Graphics, Inc. The editors were Gail Gavert and Pamela Touboul; the series editor was Hiram F. Gilbert, Ph.D.; the production supervisor was Clare Stanley; the cover designer was Andrew Thompson.

R. R. Donnelley & Sons Company was printer and binder.

This book is printed on acid-free paper.

Library of Congress Cataloging-in-Publication Data

Stringer, Janet L.
    Basic concepts in pharmacology : a student's survival guide /
Janet L. Stringer.
        p.   cm.
    Includes bibliographical references and index.
    ISBN 0-07-063165-4
    1. Pharmacology—Outlines, syllabi, etc.   2. Drugs—Outlines,
syllabi, etc.   I. Title.
    [DNLM: 1. Pharmacology.   QV 4 S918b 1995]
RM301.14.S77   1995
615′.1—dc20
DNLM/DLC
for Library of Congress   95-40461
                                                              CIP

·C O N T E N T S·

Prologue   1

CHAPTER 1   WHERE TO START   **3**

Part I   General Principles

CHAPTER 2   RECEPTOR THEORY   **9**

Agonists   9
Efficacy and Potency   10
Therapeutic Index   12
Antagonists   13

**CHAPTER 3   ABSORPTION, DISTRIBUTION,
AND CLEARANCE**   **15**

First Pass Effect   15
Drugs Crossing Membranes   16
Bioavailability   18
Total Body Clearance   19

CHAPTER 4   PHARMACOKINETICS   **21**

Volume of Distribution   21
First-Order Kinetics   23
Zero-Order Kinetics   25
Steady-State Concentration   27
Time Needed to Reach Steady-State   28
Dosing Schedules   29
Loading Dose   30

**CHAPTER 5   DRUG METABOLISM AND
RENAL ELIMINATION**   **33**

Liver Metabolism   33
Renal Excretion   34

Part II Autonomics

CHAPTER 6 REVIEW OF THE AUTONOMIC NERVOUS SYSTEM 37

Why Include This Material? 37
Relevant Anatomy 38
Synthesis, Storage, Release, and Removal of Transmitters 41
Receptors 42
General Rules of Innervation 44

CHAPTER 7 CHOLINERGIC AGONISTS 47

Organization of Class 47
Direct Cholinergic Agonists 49
Cholinesterase Inhibitors 50

CHAPTER 8 CHOLINERGIC ANTAGONISTS 53

Organization of Class 53
Muscarinic Antagonists 53
Ganglionic Blockers 55
Neuromuscular Blockers 56

CHAPTER 9 ADRENERGIC AGONISTS 59

Organization of Class 59
Direct-Acting Agonists 60
Dopamine 62
Indirect-Acting Agents 62
Cardiovascular Effects of Norepinephrine, Epinephrine,
    and Isoproterenol 63

CHAPTER 10 ADRENERGIC ANTAGONISTS 65

Organization of Class 65
Central Blockers 66
α-Blockers 66
β-Blockers 68
Labetalol 69

Part III   Drugs That Affect the Cardiovascular System

CHAPTER 15 DRUGS THAT AFFECT THE BLOOD 103

Organization of Class 103
Anticoagulants 105
Antiplatelet Agents 108
Thrombolytic or Fibrinolytic Drugs 109
Antianemia Drugs 110

CHAPTER 16 LIPID-LOWERING DRUGS 113

Organization of Class 113
Some Additional Explanation of Mechanisms 114

Part IV Drugs Acting on the Central Nervous System

CHAPTER 17 DRUGS USED IN PARKINSON'S DISEASE 119

Class Organization 119
Dopamine Replacement Therapy 120
Dopamine Agonist Therapy 121
Anticholinergic Therapy 122

CHAPTER 18 ANXIOLYTIC AND HYPNOTIC DRUGS 123

Tolerance and Dependence 123
Class Organization 124
Barbiturates 125
Benzodiazepines 127
Other Drugs 130

CHAPTER 19 ANTIDEPRESSANTS AND LITHIUM (DRUGS USED TO TREAT MOOD DISORDERS) 131

Class Organization 131
Heterocyclics 132
Serotonin-Specific Reuptake Inhibitors (SSRIs) 133
Monoamine Oxidase (MAO) Inhibitors 134
Lithium 135

CHAPTER 20   ANTIPSYCHOTICS, OR NEUROLEPTICS — 137

Class Organization — 137
"Typical" Antipsychotics — 138
"Atypical" Antipsychotics — 140

CHAPTER 21   ANTIEPILEPTIC DRUGS — 143

Class Organization — 143
Important Details About the Four Most Important Drugs — 145
Other Drugs to Consider — 146

CHAPTER 22   NARCOTICS (OPIATES) — 149

Class Organization — 149
The Actions of Morphine and, by Association, All the Other Agonists — 151
Important Distinguishing Features of Some Agonists — 152
Opioid Antagonists — 153
Opioid Agonist–Antagonists — 154

CHAPTER 23   GENERAL ANESTHETICS — 155

Class Organization — 155
Uptake and Distribution of Inhalational Anesthetics — 156
Elimination of Inhalational Anesthetics — 157
Potency of General Anesthetics — 158
Specific Gases and Volatile Liquids — 158
Specific Intravenous Agents — 160

CHAPTER 24   LOCAL ANESTHETICS — 161

Class Organization — 161
Mechanism of Action — 162
Special Features about Individual Agents — 163

Part V   Chemotherapeutic Agents

CHAPTER 25   INTRODUCTION TO CHEMOTHERAPY — 167

Approach to the Antimicrobials — 167
General Principles of Therapy — 168

Definitions   169
Big Concepts to Understand   169
Classification of Antimicrobials   172

CHAPTER 26   INHIBITORS OF CELL WALL SYNTHESIS   **173**

Features Common to *All* of the Drugs in This Group   173
β-Lactams   174
Polypeptides   179

CHAPTER 27   PROTEIN SYNTHESIS INHIBITORS   **181**

General Features of the Protein Synthesis Inhibitors   181
Aminoglycosides   182
Tetracyclines   184
Macrolides   185
Chloramphenicol   186
Clindamycin   187

CHAPTER 28   FOLATE ANTAGONISTS (SULFONAMIDES AND TRIMETHOPRIM)   **189**

Mechanism of Action   189
Selected Features   190

CHAPTER 29   QUINOLONES AND URINARY TRACT ANTISEPTICS   **191**

Drugs in This Group   191
Quinolones   192
Nitrofurantoin   193
Methenamine   193

CHAPTER 30   DRUGS USED TO TREAT TUBERCULOSIS AND LEPROSY   **195**

Class Organization   195
Isoniazid   196
Rifampin   197
Ethambutol   198
Pyrazinamide   198
Dapsone and the Treatment of Leprosy   198

CHAPTER 31   ANTIFUNGAL DRUGS   201

Class Organization   201
Polyene Antifungals   203
Azole Antifungals   203
Flucytosine   204
Griseofulvin   205
Nystatin   206

CHAPTER 32   ANTHELMINTICS   207

Class Organization   207
Treatment of Cestodes and Trematodes   208
Treatment of Nematodes   209
Treatment of Filaria   209

CHAPTER 33   ANTIVIRAL AGENTS   211

Class Organization   211
Special Features About Some of the Drugs   212

CHAPTER 34   ANTIPROTOZOAL DRUGS   215

Class Organization   215
Special Features About Some of the Drugs   216
Antimalarial Agents   217
Therapeutic Considerations   218
Special Features of Some Antimalarials   219

CHAPTER 35   ANTICANCER DRUGS   221

Organization of Class   221
Terminology and General Principles of Therapy   223
Adverse Effects   225
Alkylating Agents   228
Antimetabolites   229
Antibiotics and Other Natural Products   230
Hormonal Agents   232
Miscellaneous Agents   233
Immunomodulating Agents   233
Cellular Growth Factors   234

Part VI   Drugs That Affect the Endocrine System

CHAPTER 36   ADRENOCORTICAL HORMONES   237

Organization of Class   237
Glucocorticoids   240
Mineralocorticoids   241
Inhibitors of Adrenocorticoid Synthesis   241

CHAPTER 37   SEX STEROIDS   243

Organization of Class   243
Estrogens   245
Antiestrogens   246
Progestins   246
Antiprogestins   247
Oral Contraceptives   247
Androgens   248
Antiandrogens   249

CHAPTER 38   THYROID AND ANTITHYROID DRUGS   251

Organization of Class   251
Thyroid Replacement Therapy   252
Drugs That Are Thyroid Downers   253

CHAPTER 39   INSULIN, GLUCAGON, AND ORAL HYPOGLYCEMIC DRUGS   255

Organization of Class   255
Insulin   256
Oral Hypoglycemic Agents   257

Part VII   Miscellaneous Drugs

CHAPTER 40   HISTAMINE AND ANTIHISTAMINES   261

Organization of Class   261
H_1 Receptor Antagonists   262

CHAPTER 41   RESPIRATORY DRUGS 265

Organization of Class 265
β Agonists 266
Methylxanthines 266
Cholinergic Antagonists 267
Cromolyn 267

CHAPTER 42   DRUGS THAT AFFECT THE GI TRACT 269

Organization of Class 269
Antiulcer Drugs 269
Antidiarrheals 271
Pharmacological Treatment of Constipation 272
Inflammatory Bowel Disease 272
Dissolution of Gallstones 273

CHAPTER 43   NON-NARCOTIC ANALGESICS AND ANTI-INFLAMMATORY DRUGS 275

Organization of Class 275
NSAIDs 276
Salicylates, Including Aspirin 277
Acetaminophen 279
Gold Preparations 279
Antigout Agents 280

CHAPTER 44   IMMUNOSUPPRESSIVES 283

Organization of Class 283
Cyclosporine 283
Cytotoxic Drugs 284

CHAPTER 45   VITAMINS 285

Organization of Class 285
Fat-Soluble Vitamins 286
Water-Soluble Vitamins 286

Index 289

· P R O L O G U E ·

Basic Concepts in Pharmacology: A Student's Survival Guide is not a conventional review book for pharmacology. It is a book that will help you organize your attack on the hundreds of drugs covered in pharmacology classes today. Hopefully, using this book will minimize the stress that most students feel when they count up the number of drugs that they are expected to memorize.

We surveyed first- and second-year medical students at a national meeting. We asked what areas of pharmacology they found particularly difficult conceptually. Number one was antiarrhythmics, followed by cardiovascular drugs in general, and then antibiotics. However, it is clear from the comments that the number of drugs in a particular class was often overwhelming.

Because this is not a review book, I will not be covering each and every drug available in the market. Instead, I will try to provide a way to organize and condense the amount of material that needs to be memorized. In addition, some concepts and definitions will be explained. For each group of drugs I will point out ways to study and how to determine the most important information. Along the way we will need to review some biochemistry and physiology, reinforcing previously learned concepts.

1

· C H A P T E R · 1 ·

WHERE TO START

·

> You cannot possibly learn everything about every drug available.

Remember that you are human. While many pharmacology students are able to memorize an incredible amount of useful and useless information, there is a limit to what even the best students can learn. Therefore, you must try to organize the material in such a way that you memorize the least amount of material necessary. You need to get the most bang for your buck, or most facts learned for each hour of time spent. Usually this means grouping drugs and making associations.

> New drugs will be introduced during your lifetime and even during your training, so develop a flexible framework for drug information.

The best approach is to learn the drugs by class. If you know the characteristics of angiotensin-converting enzyme inhibitors (Chap. 11), then when a new one is marketed you will have a framework for comparison.

Many students try to memorize everything about a drug and end up remembering the most trivial facts and forgetting the most important. Often, from your perspective it is very difficult to know what is most important and what can be skipped or forgotten to make room for other facts.

3

This is a result of the way most textbooks are organized. They give general information about the pathophysiology or the drug class and then provide details about each individual agent in the class. This is a very efficient way to be thorough and it is very useful when you need to go back and look up a detail about a drug. It is not as useful, however, for the beginning student who must start from scratch to learn the information.

To help you decide what is the most important information, I have developed a trivia sorter.

This generic trivia sorter will not work for all drug classes. Therefore, for each class I will indicate the way I have organized my attack on the drugs in that group. For example, the mechanism of action of the anti-epileptic drugs is not clear, so you will have to skip No. 1 and go to No. 2. The antiarrythmics are classified and grouped according to their mechanism of action, so that should be the No. 1 item you learn.

You can determine your own trivia level: I would suggest at least down through number 6. This book is designed to help you through the first 6 layers of material. If you have the time and inclination to get into more trivial details you will need to consult your favorite textbook.

Because the DRUG OF CHOICE is often very important to know, these will be presented in a box throughout the book. However, these are subject to change, so you should confirm that that drug is still the drug of choice during class or from your textbook. Fatal side effects, even if rare, are important to know for your patients sake. I will try to point out some, but others may come up in class or in your book. If so, make a note to learn them.

GENERIC TRIVIA SORTER
1. The mechanism of action for the class of drug
2. Kinetics properties, major side effects or major actions that are common to all drugs in this class
3. Is/are the drug(s) the DRUG OF CHOICE for something?
4. Name recognition: what drugs are in this class?
5. Unique features about single drugs in the class
6. Are there any side effects (rare or not) that may be FATAL?
7. Drug interactions
8. Rare side effects or actions that are common to all drugs in the class
9. Rare side effects or actions for single drugs in the class
10. Percentage of drug that is metabolized versus renal excretion
11. Half-life of each drug in the class
12. Teratogenicity of each drug in the class
13. Structure of each drug in the class

The idea of name recognition is a bit different. This comes about from the experience of medical students, including myself, who sat down to take an exam in pharmacology, then got to a question that asked about a drug that looked unfamiliar. Most of the time the question was missed, but if the drug class could have been identified, then the question was simple. I recommend to students who are having trouble with this to make flash cards (or lists) with only the drug name on one side and the drug class on the other side. Skip the easy ones. Quiz yourself during breakfast or during breaks between classes. As you learn the drugs, take them off your list or remove the card from the stack. Occasionally add back in all the names. If you only get a few more questions right on your exam or the boards, or have to look up one less drug after rounds, the few minutes that this takes will have been worth it.

Because students are only expected to know generic names of drugs, only generic names will be used throughout this text. Trade names are given in the index.

Information in these boxes is key. If you know the information in the box skip on to the next one. If you don't know the information read the following text.

This book is organized so that the reader can read the highlights and decide whether or not to read the more detailed description. If you know the material and understand the concept, don't waste your time with the explanation. This book is to help you organize your study and waste less time on less important trivia, so approach the book the same way.

Some drug names appear in capital letters in the text. These are the drug names that are the most important to know (a somewhat arbitrary decision). If you only have time and energy to learn three names in a particular drug class, learn the ones that appear in capital letters.

· P A R T · I ·

GENERAL PRINCIPLES

·

· C H A P T E R · 2 ·

RECEPTOR THEORY

·

Agonists

Efficacy and Potency

Therapeutic Index

Antagonists

· · · · · · · · · · · ·

AGONISTS

A drug receptor is a specialized target macromolecule that binds a drug and mediates its pharmacological action. These receptors may be enzymes, nucleic acids, or specialized membrane-bound proteins. The formation of the drug–receptor complex leads to a biological response. The magnitude of the response is proportional to the number of drug–receptor complexes. A common way to present the relationship between the drug concentration and biological response is a concentration– or dose–response curve (Fig. 2-1). You will see both dose–response curves and concentration-response curves. Since the biological effect is more closely related to the plasma concentration than to the dose, I will show concentration-response curves in this text.

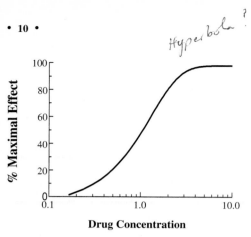

Hyperbola ?

Figure 2-1
In a concentration–response curve, the concentration of the drug is plotted against the percent maximal effect. Notice that the drug concentration is plotted on a log scale. In this graph the drug is a full agonist—the effect reaches 100 percent of the maximum that is possible.

An agonist is a compound that binds to a receptor and produces the biological response.

An agonist can be a drug or the endogenous ligand for the receptor. Increasing concentrations of the agonist will increase the biological response until either no more receptors are available for the agonist to bind or a maximal response has been reached.

A partial agonist produces the biological response, but cannot produce 100 percent of the biological response even at very high doses.

Partial agonists are compared to full agonists (Fig. 2-2).

EFFICACY AND POTENCY

Efficacy and *potency* are terms that students sometimes confuse. These terms are used for comparisons between drugs.

Efficacy is the maximal response that a drug can produce. Potency is a measure of the dose that is required to produce a response.

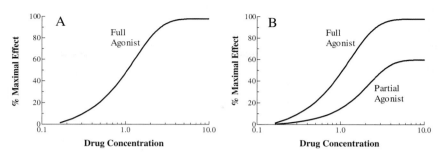

Figure 2-2
In *A*, the concentration–response curve for a full agonist is presented. The drug can produce a maximal effect. In *B*, the concentration–response curve for a partial agonist is also shown. In this case, the partial agonist is only able to produce 60 percent of the maximal response.

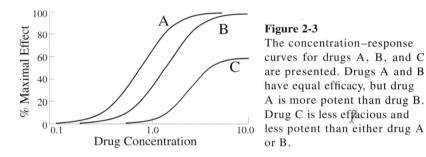

Figure 2-3
The concentration–response curves for drugs A, B, and C are presented. Drugs A and B have equal efficacy, but drug A is more potent than drug B. Drug C is less efficacious and less potent than either drug A or B.

For example: one drug (drug A) produces complete eradication of premature ventricular contractions (PVCs) at a dose of 10 mg. A second drug (drug B) produces complete eradication of PVCs at a dose of 20 mg. Therefore, both drugs have the same efficacy (complete eradication of PVCs), but drug A is more potent than drug B. It takes less milligrams of drug A to produce the same effect. A third drug (drug C) can only produce a 60 percent reduction in the PVCs and it takes a dose of 50 mg to achieve that effect. Therefore, drug C has less efficacy and potency in the reduction of PVCs as compared with drug A or drug B.

Potency and efficacy are usually shown graphically (Fig. 2-3).

Potency is often expressed as the dose of drug required to achieve 50 percent of the desired therapeutic effect. This is the ED_{50} (effective dose).

THERAPEUTIC INDEX

> Therapeutic index is a measure of drug safety. A drug with a larger therapeutic index is safer than one with a low therapeutic index.

The above statement is true no matter what book you consult. The therapeutic index is a definition that sometimes varies, depending on the book consulted.

Usually:

$$\text{therapeutic index} = \frac{LD_{50}}{ED_{50}}$$

The LD_{50} is the dose the kills 50 percent of the animals that received it.

This is somewhat different from the therapeutic window. The therapeutic index is determined from the ED_{50} and the LD_{50}. The therapeutic window compares the range of effective drug concentration to the safety of the drug. In the example in Fig. 2-4, notice that the drug in graph A has a much wider therapeutic window than the drug in graph B, even though both drugs have the same therapeutic index.

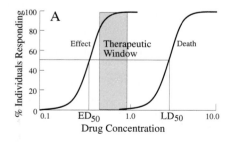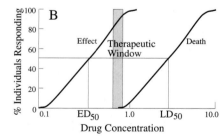

Figure 2-4

Instead of concentration–response curves, here the percentage of individuals responding is graphed against the drug concentration. In both graphs, the drugs have the same therapeutic index. Because of the different slopes of the curves, however, the drug in A has a wider therapeutic window than the drug in B.

ANTAGONISTS

> Antagonists block or reverse the effect of agonists. They have no effect of their own.

Antagonists can block the effect of agonists, or they can reverse the effect of the agonist. Binding of the antagonist to the receptor does not produce a biological effect. We will see instances where the administration of an antagonist has an effect on blood pressure. In this case the agonist is produced by the autonomic nervous system and is not administered exogenously. Another example of an antagonist is naloxone, an opioid antagonist (Chap. 22). Naloxone has no effect of its own, but will completely reverse the effects of any opioid agonist that has been administered.

> Competitive antagonists make the agonist appear less potent.

Since the antagonists theoretically have no effect of their own, we need to consider their effect on the agonist. In the graph (Fig. 2-5) we determined the biological effect produced by a series of concentrations of agonist. We then repeated the same experiment in the presence of a fixed concentration of antagonist. This shifted the curve to the right, making the agonist appear less potent.

This is easy to remember and understand. These antagonists are competitive, that is, they compete for the same site on the receptor that the agonist wants. If the agonist wins, a response is produced. If the antagonist

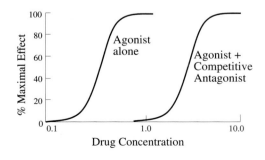

Figure 2-5
In this graph the concentration–response curve for an agonist alone is presented. When the effect of the agonist is tested in the presence of a fixed concentration of a competitive antagonist, the agonist appears less potent. The same maximal effect is achieved, but it takes higher doses.

wins, no response is produced. As we increase the concentration of agonist, we increase the odds that an agonist molecule will win the receptor spot and produce an effect. At high enough agonist concentration the poor antagonist doesn't have a chance at the receptor; it is too outnumbered.

A noncompetitive antagonist reduces the maximal response that the agonist can produce.

Noncompetitive antagonists bind to the receptor at a site different from the agonist and either prevent agonist binding or prevent the agonist effect (Fig. 2-6).

Let us try our experiment again. We determine the biological effect produced by increasing concentrations of agonist. We plot the results as shown in Fig. 2.5). We repeat these measurements in the presence of a fixed concentration of antagonist. The antagonist binds to its very own site and blocks the effect of the agonist. Increasing concentrations of agonist cannot overcome this blockade. Therefore, the maximal biological response produced by the agonist appears to have decreased because of our addition of the noncompetitive antagonist.

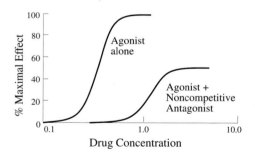

Figure 2-6
The concentration–response curve for the same agonist alone is presented. Then, the activity of the agonist is tested in the presence of a fixed concentration of noncompetitive antagonist. In this instance the maximal response is reduced.

ABSORPTION, DISTRIBUTION AND CLEARANCE

·

First-Pass Effect

Drugs Crossing Membranes

Bioavailability

Total Body Clearance

· · · · · · · · · · · ·

FIRST PASS EFFECT

> The liver is a metabolic machine and often inactivates drugs on their way from the GI tract to the body. This is called the *first-pass effect.*

Orally administered drugs are absorbed from the GI tract. The blood from the GI tract then travels through the liver—the great chemical plant in the body. Many drugs that undergo liver metabolism will be extensively metabolized during this passage from the GI tract to the body. This effect of liver metabolism is called the first-pass effect.

DRUGS CROSSING MEMBRANES

The are a number of useful routes of drug administration, but almost all require that the drug cross a biological membrane to reach its site of action.

Drugs cross membranes by:
  Passive diffusion
  Active transport

This is somewhat simplified, but a useful starting point. Passive diffusion requires a concentration gradient across the membrane. The vast majority of drugs gain access to their site of action by this method. Water-soluble drugs can penetrate the cell membrane through aqueous channels. More commonly, lipid-soluble drugs just move through the membrane.

A drug tends to pass through membranes if it is uncharged.

Uncharged drugs are more lipid soluble than charged drugs. In addition, many drugs are weak acids or weak bases.

For a weak acid, when the pH is less than the pK, the protonated form (un-ionized) predominates. When the pH is greater than the pK, the unprotonated (ionized) form predominates.

$$HA \rightleftharpoons H^+ + A^-$$

Weak acids are hydrogen ion donors; they are happy to give up a hydrogen ion and become charged. If you have trouble remembering whether they become charged or uncharged after donating their hydrogen ion, think of a strong acid, such as HCl. Of course, you know that when you put HCl into water it immediately turns into H^+ and Cl^-. Use this to remember that weak acids donate a hydrogen ion and become charged.

Remember the pK? That is the equilibrium constant (of course, the p means we've taken the log of the equilibrium constant). When the pH is equal to the pK, the above equation is balanced; there are equal amounts of weak acid in the ionized and un-ionized forms. If we decrease the pH by adding more H^+, we will drive the equilibrium for the weak acid more to the left, which is the un-ionized (uncharged) form.

If we take away H^+, making the pH higher, we will drive the equilibrium towards the right. This increases the concentration of the ionized form of the weak acid (Fig. 3-1).

For a weak base, when the pH is less than the pK, the ionized form (protonated) predominates. When the pH is greater than the pK, the unprotonated (un-ionized) form predominates.

Weak bases are the opposite of weak acids. A weak base is a hydrogen ion acceptor. It sits around in solution doing just fine, but if a loose hydrogen ion asks to join it, it may say yes. If it accepts the hydrogen ion, then it becomes charged.

$$B + H^+ \rightleftharpoons BH^+$$

Adding H^+ to lower the pH will drive the equilibrium to the right towards the protonated (charged) form. Removing H^+ to raise the pH will drive the equilibrium to the left towards the uncharged (unprotonated) form of the base (Fig. 3-2).

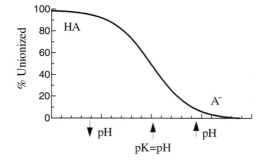

Figure 3-1
The relationship between the pH and the degree of ionization of a weak acid is presented. When the pH is above the pK for the acid, the charged form of the acid predominates.

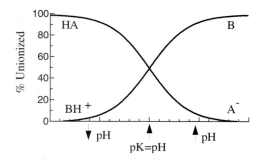

Figure 3-2
 In this graph the effect of pH on the degree of ionization of both a weak acid and a weak base is presented.

In the stomach (pH 2), weak acids are uncharged and will be absorbed into the bloodstream, while weak bases are charged and will remain in the GI tract.

To test your understanding of this, try out these questions. The answers appear at the bottom of the page.*

1. In the intestine (pH 8.0), which will be better absorbed, a weak acid (pK 6.8) or a weak base (pK 7.1)?
2. If we alkalinize the urine to a pH of 7.8, will a lower or higher percentage of a weak acid (pK 7.1) be ionized, compared to when the urine pH was 7.2?

BIOAVAILABILITY

Bioavailability is the amount of drug that is absorbed after administration by route X compared with the amount of drug that is absorbed after intravenous administration. X is any route of drug administration other than intravenous.

An example for oral administration: you are testing a compound for clinical trials. You have tentatively named the drug Newdrug. Newdrug is administered orally and plasma levels determine that only 75 percent of the oral dose reaches the circulation. Compared with intravenous administra-

*(1) Base. (2) Higher, more weak acid will be ionized the more the pH exceeds the pK.

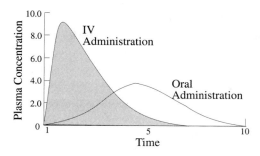

Figure 3-3
The plasma concentration is plotted against time and the area under the curve is an indication of bioavailability. Here a drug is given orally and compared with the intravenous route of administration.

tion where 100 percent of the dose reaches the circulation, the bioavailability of Newdrug is 0.75 or 75 percent. In the case of hypothetical Newdrug, you discover that some of the drug is inactivated by the acid in the stomach. You redesign the pill with a coating that is stable in acid, but dissolves in the more basic pH of the small intestine. The bioavailability of the drug increases to 95 percent. You make millions on the sales of Newdrug.

Bioavailability is the area under the curve (AUC) when plotting the plasma concentration of a drug versus the time after single-dose administration (Fig. 3-3).

$$\text{Bioavailability} = \frac{\text{AUC}_{oral}}{\text{AUC}_{iv}}$$

TOTAL BODY CLEARANCE

Clearance is a term that indicates the rate at which a drug is cleared from the body. It is defined as the volume of plasma from which all drug is removed in a given time. This gives units for clearance of volume/time.

Clearance is an odd term, mostly because of its units. It is not intuitive. Try this out as a way to remember this.

Let's say we have 1 liter of water that contains 1000 mg of drug (Fig. 3-4). The concentration is 1 mg/ml. One hour later, 100 mg of drug have been removed. That leaves 900 mg of drug in the water. We then divide the

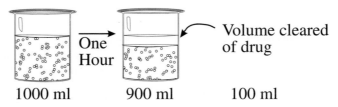

1000 ml   **900 ml**   **100 ml**

Figure 3-4
On the left is a beaker containing 1000 ml of water and a certain concentration of a drug. After 1 hour, we find the same concentration of the drug in only 900 ml of water. The 100 ml of water that has been cleared of drug represents the clearance in one hour. This gives us units of volume per unit time for clearance.

water into 2 compartments. One compartment contains 1 mg/ml of our drug and the other compartment contains no drug. In this example, the drug-containing compartment would be 900 ml of water and the empty compartment would be 100 ml. This 100 ml of water represents the amount of water that is cleared of drug in 1 hour. This volume is the clearance.
    A more official definition is the following equation:

$$\text{clearance} = \frac{\text{rate of removal of drug (mg/min)}}{\text{plasma concentration of drug (mg/ml)}}$$

    Notice that this gives you units of ml/min, or volume per unit time.

Total body clearance is the sum of the clearances from the various metabolizing and eliminating organs.

PHARMACOKINETICS

·

Volume of distribution

First-Order kinetics

Zero-Order kinetics

Steady-State concentration

Time Needed to Reach Steady-State

Dosing Schedules

Loading Dose

·   ·   ·   ·   ·   ·   ·   ·   ·   ·   ·   ·

Pharmacokinetics is the mathematical description of the rate and extent of uptake, distribution, and elimination of drugs in the body.

VOLUME OF DISTRIBUTION

Volume of distribution is a definition and it does not correspond to any real volume. It assumes that the drug is evenly distributed and that metabolism or elimination has not taken place.

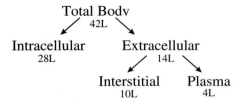

Total Body
42L

Intracellular   Extracellular
28L   14L

Interstitial   Plasma
10L   4L

Figure 4-1
The various body fluid compartments for your standard
70-kg man are illustrated in
this figure. Do you know any-
one that is 70 kg?

$$\text{Volume of distribution } (V_D) = \frac{\text{dose (mg)}}{\text{plasma concentration (mg/ml)}}$$

This is very easy to remember. Take 1000 mg of sugar and dissolve it into a beaker of water. After it has dissolved, take a sample of water (say 10 ml) and determine the concentration of sugar in that sample (say 1 mg/ml). From this you can calculate the volume of water in which the sugar was dissolved.

$$\frac{1 \text{ mg}}{\text{ml}} = \frac{1000 \text{ mg}}{\text{volume of water}}$$

$$\text{volume of water} = \frac{1000 \text{ mg}}{1 \text{ mg/ml}} = 1{,}000 \text{ ml}$$

In this case the volume was 1000 ml or 1 liter. If you keep the units straight the equation does not need to be memorized.

Try another one. A 500-mg of Newdrug is administered to a medical student. The plasma concentration is 0.01 mg/ml. What is the volume of distribution?*

This gives a very large volume of distribution. Your selected medical student is not a huge water balloon. The only other option is that the drug is hiding somewhere in the body where it is not recorded by the plasma concentration. The drug could be very lipid soluble and stored in fat, or it could be bound to plasma proteins. This example shows that the volume of distribution is a hypothetical volume and not a real volume.

The volume of distribution gives a rough accounting of where a drug goes in the body, especially if you have a feel for the various body fluid compartments and their size (Fig. 4-1). In addition, it can be used to calculate the dose of drug needed to achieve a desired plasma concentration.

*50,000 ml or 50 liters.

FIRST-ORDER KINETICS

The order of a reaction refers to the way in which the concentration of drug or reactant influences the rate of a chemical reaction. For most drug reactions we only need consider first order and zero order.

Most drugs disappear from plasma by processes that are concentration dependent, which is first order.

With first-order elimination a constant percentage of the drug is lost per unit time. An elimination rate constant can be described.

The elimination rate constant is k_e (units are 1/time). On the log plot (Fig. 4-2), which is linear, the slope is equal to $-k_e/2.303$. The factor 2.303 converts from natural log to base 10 log units.

The half-life is the period of time required for the concentration of a drug to decrease by one-half.

The half-life is shown in Fig. 4-3

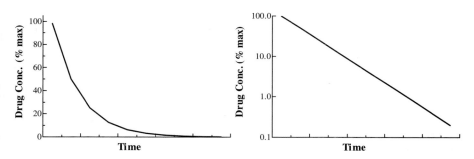

Figure 4-2
Both graphs present the elimination of a drug that follows first-order kinetics. On the left, the y-axis is a linear scale, while on the right, the y-axis is a log scale. Notice that first-order reactions are linear when graphed on the log scale.

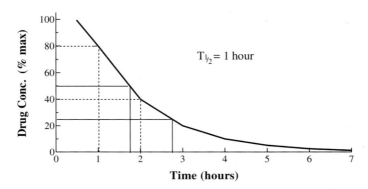

Figure 4-3
The determiniation of the half-life of a drug with first-order kinetics is illustrated. The drug concentration is graphed against time. The time it takes for the concentration to decrease by 50 percent as indicated in 2 places on the curve. The half-life is the same for both determinations.

The half-life is constant and related to k_e for drugs that have first-order kinetics.

$$t_{1/2} = \frac{0.693}{k_e}$$

A first-order elimination rate equals

rate constant $\times$ plasma concentration $\times$ volume of distribution
$= k$ (1/min) $\times C_p$ (mg/ml) $\times V_D$ (ml) $=$ mg/min

---

Clearance of a drug is different from the elimination rate.

Remember clearance? That's the volume of fluid cleared of a drug per unit time. The elimination rate is the rate of removal of drug in units of weight per unit time.

$$\text{Clearance} = \frac{\text{rate of removal of drug (mg/min)}}{\text{plasma concentration of drug (mg/ml)}} = \text{ml/min}$$

For drugs with first-order kinetics, the V_D, $t_{1/2}$, k_e, and clearance are all interrelated.

You can do all kinds of juggling with these equations. For example, let's take the equation for clearance.

$$\text{Clearance} = \frac{\text{elimination rate}}{\text{plasma concentration}}$$

Now substitute in the first order elimination rate equation.

$$\text{Clearance} = \frac{k \times C_p \times V_D}{C_p}$$
$$\text{Clearance} = k \times V_D$$

Therefore, clearance is directly related to the elimination rate constant and the volume of distribution. But remember that

$$t_{1/2} = \frac{0.693}{k_e}$$
$$\text{or } k_e = \frac{0.693}{t_{1/2}}$$

Therefore,

$$\text{clearance} = \frac{0.693}{t_{1/2}} \times V_D$$

It should be clear from this that for drugs that have first-order kinetics, the V_D, $t_{1/2}$, k_e, and clearance are all interconnected.

ZERO-ORDER KINETICS

Drugs that saturate routes of elimination will disappear from plasma in a nonconcentration-dependent manner, which is zero order.

Metabolism in the liver, which involves specific enzymes, is one of the most important factors that contribute to a drug having zero-order kinetics. The most common examples of drugs that have zero-order kinetics are aspirin, phenytoin and ethanol. Many drugs will show zero-order kinetics at high, or toxic, concentrations.

For drugs with zero-order kinetics, a constant amount of drug is lost per unit time.

The half-life is not constant for zero-order reactions, but depends on the concentration.

The higher the concentration, the longer the half-life. This is illustrated in Fig. 4-4 above. Because the $t_{1/2}$ changes as the drug concentration declines, the zero-order half-life has little practical significance.

Zero-order kinetics is also known as nonlinear or dose-dependent.

You will see these terms used interchangeably in the medical literature.

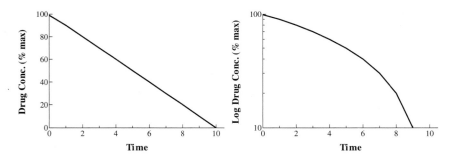

Figure 4-4
A drug showing zero-order elimination kinetics is illustrated here. On the left, the drug concentration is plotted on a linear scale, and on the right, on a log scale. Notice that drugs with zero-order kinetics show a linear plot on the linear scale. Try calculating the half-life of this drug in at least two different places. Do you get the same half-life?

STEADY-STATE CONCENTRATION

> With multiple dosing or a continuous infusion, drug will accumulate until the amount administrated per unit time is equal to the amount eliminated per unit time. The plasma concentration at this point is called the *steady-state concentration* (C_{ss}).

Rarely are drugs given as a single dose. Normally, repeated doses are given and sometimes drugs are given as a continuous intravenous infusion. When a drug is given as a continuous infusion it will increase in concentration in the blood until the rate of elimination is equal to the infusion rate. At this point the amount administered per unit time is equal to the amount excreted. The plasma concentration at this point is called the concentration at steady-state, or C_{ss} (Fig. 4-5).

Let's start with a patient that has no drug on board. Start an IV infusion at 100 mg/kg. At first the plasma level will be low and the infusion rate will be greater than the elimination rate. The plasma level will rise relatively quickly. Remember that the elimination rate is proportional to the plasma concentration of the drug, so as the concentration rises so does the elimination rate. The rate of increase in the plasma level will slow as the concentration rises. At steady-state, the infusion rate and the elimination rate are equal.

For an IV infusion,

$$C_{ss} = \frac{\text{infusion rate (mg/min)}}{\text{clearance (ml/min)}} = \text{mg/ml}$$

Notice the direct relationship between C_{ss} and the infusion rate (assuming clearance is constant). If we double the infusion rate, the C_{ss} doubles.

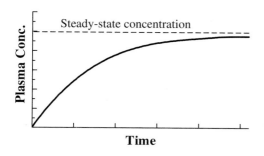

Time

Figure 4-5
A continuous intravenous infusion of a drug was started at the beginning of the graph. The concentration of the drug in the plasma was followed over time. When the amount delivered in a unit of time is equal to the amount eliminated in the same time unit, the plasma concentration is said to have reached steady-state.

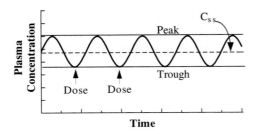

Figure 4-6
This graph shows the change
in concentration with repeated
doses. Peak and trough levels
are indicated, as well as the
steady-state concentration (or
average concentration).

There is also a concentration at steady-state for repeated doses. Some books will call this an average concentration (C_{av}). With multiple dosing schedules we normally assume that early doses of the drug do not affect the pharmacokinetics of subsequent doses. Generally, we also give equal doses at equal time intervals.

> Repeated dosing is associated with peak and trough plasma concentrations.

With repeated dosing the concentration fluctuates around a mean (steady-state value) with peak and trough values. Here steady-state is achieved when the dose administered and the amount eliminated in a given dosing interval is the same (Fig. 4-6).

TIME NEEDED TO REACH STEADY-STATE

The discussion above was about the concentration at steady-state. Now let us consider the time it takes to reach this steady-state concentration.

> The time to reach steady-state depends *only* on the half-life of the drug. Ninety percent of steady-state is reached in 3.3 half-lives.

There is a lot of math behind these numbers, which you can read about if you want. The bottom line is that during each half-life, 50 percent of the change from the starting point to C_{ss} is achieved.

NUMBER OF HALF-LIVES	% C_{ss}
1	50
2	75
3	88
3.3	90
4	94
5	97

After one half-life, we gain 50 percent of the C_{ss}. We have 50 percent of the distance remaining. In the next half-life we will gain 50 percent of this remaining distance, or $1/2 \times 50$ percent, which is 25 percent. So after 2 half-lives we will be 75 percent of the way to steady-state. If you repeat this several times, you can generate the table above. Notice that after 5 half-lives we are still approaching steady-state.

When asked the question, How long does it take to get to steady-state? some books will accept $3.3 \times t_{1/2}$ (90 percent of C_{ss}) and others want $4 \times t_{1/2}$ and still others accept $5 \times t_{1/2}$. Check your book or lecture notes.

DOSING SCHEDULES

So, why have we gone through all of this stuff?

Most of the time we need to consistently keep a drug within certain blood levels in order to get the desired therapeutic effect. Suppose that you have an ear infection. You should take an antibiotic at a high enough dose and frequently enough so that your blood levels are high enough to kill the bacteria, but not so high that the antibiotic makes you feel worse (Fig. 4-7).

Maintaining the plasma concentration in the therapeutic range without getting into the toxic range requires adequate adjustment of the dose and dosing interval.

To determine the effect of a change in the dose schedule on the steady-state concentration, calculate the total dose received in a fixed time period (e.g., 24 hours).

The most important part of dose schedule problems is to determine the effect of the schedule change on the steady-state concentration. To do this, first pick a time interval, such as 24 or 48 hours. Calculate the total dose

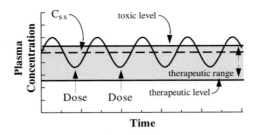

Figure 4-7
The changing plasma concentration between doses at steady-state are graphed. The lowest therapeutically effective dose is indicated (therapeutic level) as well as the dose at which the drug begins to have toxic side effects (toxic level). The plasma concentrations between the therapeutic level and the toxic level is the therapeutic range. In this example, the drug plasma concentrations were within the therapeutic range most of the time, but were reaching toxic levels at the peak concentrations.

(mg) the patient will receive in that time interval. Has this number gone up or down? If it has gone up the steady-state concentration has gone up. If it has gone down the steady-state concentration has gone down.

Doubling the frequency while halving the dose does not change the steady-state concentration.

Changing the dose interval and the dose at the same time has more complex but predictable effects.

Let us suppose that you have a patient on an antihypertensive drug. She is getting a good therapeutic effect, but shortly after each dose she has annoying toxic effects. This information tells you that the steady-state concentration is probably in the therapeutic range, but that the peak levels are in the toxic range. You wish to reduce the peak levels without decreasing the steady-state concentration. If her current dose schedule is 200 mg every 8 hours, what change in the dose schedule would you make?*

LOADING DOSE

If the half-life of a drug is relatively long, such as 6.7 days for digitoxin, it will take quite a long time for the drug concentration to reach steady-

*Answer: Keep the total dose in 24 hours constant. Divide the total dose (600 mg) into 4 separate doses during the day. The new schedule is 150 mg every 6 hours.

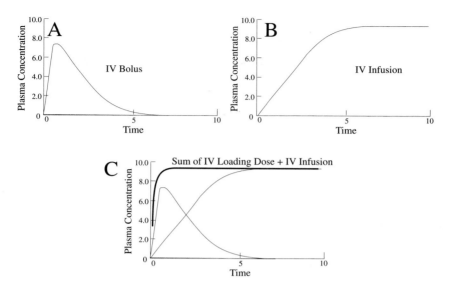

Figure 4-8
In *A*, the change in drug concentration as a function of time after an IV bolus is presented. In *B*, the change in drug concentration as a function of time after the start of a continuous IV infusion is presented. If both the bolus and the continuous infusion are given at time 0, then we see the effect of a loading dose in *C*. The IV bolus is the loading dose. See how fast the plasma concentration reaches the steady state concentration with this technique.

state (about four times the half-life). For digitoxin, this would take over 3 weeks. Sometimes the patient can't wait that long for the therapeutic effect to take place. In these instances a loading dose is used.

A *loading dose* is a single large dose of a drug that is used to get the plasma concentration to a therapeutic level more quickly than repeated smaller doses.

A single dose of a drug can be given that will result in the desired plasma concentration. This dose is called a loading dose, if it is followed by repeated doses, or continuous infusion, that will maintain the plasma concentration at that level (termed *maintenance doses*).

You can see from Fig. 4-8, as the concentration begins to decline after the loading dose, the concentration that is contributed by the continuous infusion is beginning to increase.

DRUG METABOLISM AND RENAL ELIMINATION

·

Liver Metabolism

Renal Excretion

LIVER METABOLISM

The liver is the major site for drug metabolism. The goal of metabolism is to produce metabolites that are polar, or charged, and can be eliminated by the kidney. Lipid-soluble agents are metabolized by the liver using two general sets of reactions, termed Phase I and Phase II. (Don't ask, I don't know who named them.)

> Phase I reactions frequently involve the cytochrome P-450 system. Phase II reactions are conjugations, mostly with glucuronide.

Phase I reactions convert lipophilic molecules into more polar molecules by introducing or unmasking a polar functional group, such as an −OH or $-NH_2$. Most of these reaction utilize the microsomal P-450 enzymes. A few reactions that are classified as Phase I do not.

Phase II reactions are conjugation reactions. These combine a glucuronic acid, sulfuric acid, acetic acid, or an amino acid with the drug molecule to make it more polar. The highly polar drugs can then be excreted by the kidney.

RENAL EXCRETION

Renal elimination of drugs involves three physiological processes:
  Glomerular filtration
  Proximal tubular secretion
  Distal tubular reabsorption

1. *Glomerular filtration.* Free drug flows out of the body and into the urine-to-be as part of the glomerular filtrate. Size of the molecule is the only limiting factor at this step.
2. *Proximal tubular secretion.* Some drugs are actively secreted into the proximal tubule.
3. *Distal tubular reabsorption.* Uncharged drugs may diffuse out of the kidney and escape elimination. Manipulating the pH of the urine may alter this process by changing the ionization of the weak acids and bases. This process was described in detail for passive diffusion of drugs across membranes. However, if we want excretion, we want the drug to be charged so that it is trapped in the urine and can't cross the membrane to sneak back into the body.

Reminder: When the pH is above the pK, the unprotonated forms (A^- and B) predominate. When the pH is below the pK, the protonated forms (AH and B^+) predominate.

· P A R T · I I ·

AUTONOMICS

·

REVIEW OF THE AUTONOMIC NERVOUS SYSTEM

·

Why Include this Material?

Relevant Anatomy

Synthesis, Storage, Release, and Removal of Transmitters

Receptors

General Rules of Innervation

· · · · · · · · · · · ·

WHY INCLUDE THIS MATERIAL?

Why include a review of the autonomic nervous system in a book on pharmacology? The main reason is that autonomic pharmacology is easiest if you have an understanding of the anatomy and physiology of the autonomic nervous system. Therefore, a quick review of the autonomic nervous system should simplify the pharmacology. Please keep in mind that autonomic pharmacology is often the most emphasized section of pharmacology on board exams. It is not uncommon to see graphs of changes in blood pressure, heart rate, and peripheral vascular resistance after administration of one or more of these drugs. In addition, autonomic pharmacology forms a basis for cardiovascular and central nervous system pharmacology. So, learning the autonomics well will save you time and energy later on.

Hopefully you learned the anatomy and physiology of the autonomic nervous system in your anatomy and physiology classes. So let us begin with a quiz to see how much you remember and then move on to a review of the pertinent facts.

Fill in the blanks in the following sentences. If you can do so easily, you are in great shape and should skip the rest of this chapter.*

1. All preganglionic fibers of the autonomic nervous system use the neurotransmitter _____.
2. The major neurotransmitter for sympathetic postganglionic fibers is _____.
3. Stimulation of sympathetic innervation to the eye causes contraction of the _____ and, therefore, _____ of the pupil.
4. The rate-limiting step in the synthesis of norepinephrine is _____.
5. The major pathway for the termination of the action of norepinephrine is _____.
6. The actions of acetylcholine released from parasympathetic fibers in viscera are mediated by _____ receptors.
7. Adrenergic receptors in the heart are predominantly _____.
8. Stimulation of α_1 receptors causes predominantly _____ of blood vessels.
9. Stimulation of the sympathetic nervous system causes _____ in gluconeogenesis and glycogenolysis.
10. Stimulation of the β_2 receptor in the pregnant uterus causes _____ of the smooth muscle.

Some of those sentences were pretty picky. So if you got them all you are doing really great. If you got most you are doing really well. If you only got a few, please read on.

RELEVANT ANATOMY

The nervous system is divided into parts: the central nervous system and the peripheral nervous system (Fig. 6-1). The central nervous system contains the brain and spinal cord. The peripheral nervous system is everything else, including all of the sensory information going to the brain and all the information flowing out of the brain. The peripheral nervous system

*Answers: (1) acetylcholine; (2) norepinephrine; (3) radial; dilation; (4) the formation of DOPA by tyrosine β-hydroxylase; (5) reuptake; (6) muscarinic; (7) β_1; (8) constriction; (9) an increase; (10) relaxation.

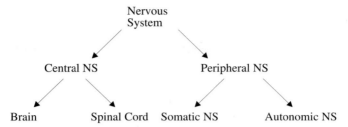

Figure 6-1
The scheme shows the major divisions of the nervous system.

is divided into two main parts: the somatic and autonomic. The somatic nervous system is mainly the motor system, which includes all of the nerves to the muscles. The autonomic nervous system is the other part (and is the part we are interested in).

The autonomic nervous system is responsible for maintaining the internal environment of the body (homeostasis).

Knowing the role of the autonomic nervous system in homeostasis makes it easy to remember the target organs. Clearly, the cardiovascular system needs regulation, but also the smooth muscle of the GI tract and the various glands throughout the body need to be constantly monitored.

Let us consider some points that are true about the *entire* autonomic nervous system, before we break it down into parts.

Within the autonomic nervous system, two neurons are required to reach the target organ: a preganglionic neuron and a postganglionic neuron.

The preganglionic neuron originates in the central nervous system. It synapses on the postganglionic neuron, whose cell body is located in auto-nomic ganglia. Simple enough!

All preganglionic neurons release acetylcholine as their transmitter. The acetylcholine binds to nicotinic receptors on the postganglionic cell.

We'll get back to the transmitter and receptors in more detail later. This is just a general rule.

The autonomic nervous system is divided into the sympathetic and parasympathetic systems (Fig. 6-2). The sympathetic system is catabolic, meaning that it burns energy. It is the one involved in the fight-or-flight response. If you remember this, most of the effects of the sympathetic nervous system "make sense." The sympathetic nervous system is also called the thoracolumbar system, since the ganglia are located lateral to the vertebral column in the thoracic and lumber regions. Since the ganglia are fixed along the back, the postganglionic fibers can be quite long. Within the sympathetic system the preganglionic axons form synapses with many post-ganglionic cells, giving this system a widespread action. Note that this is consistent with the fight-or-flight response.

The parasympathetic system is anabolic, meaning that it tries to conserve energy. It is sometimes called the craniosacral system. The pre-ganglionic neurons are found in the brainstem and in the sacral region of the spinal cord. In the parasympathetic system the ganglia are located closer to the target organs (they are not fixed along the vertebral column). Therefore, the preganglionic axons tend to be long and the postganglionic fibers are shorter. Within the parasympathetic system one presynaptic axon tends to synapse with only one or two postganglionic cells, giving the parasympathetic system a more localized action.

All of the parasympathetic postganglionic fibers release acetylcholine. At the target organ acetylcholine interacts with muscarinic receptors.

The key word above is ALL. More on the muscarinic receptors later.

Most of the sympathetic postganglionic fibers release norepineph-rine. At the target organ norepinephrine interacts with a variety of receptors.

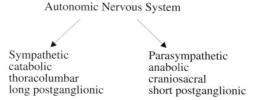

Autonomic Nervous System

Sympathetic
catabolic
thoracolumbar
long postganglionic

Parasympathetic
anabolic
craniosacral
short postganglionic

Figure 6-2
 The two divisions of the autonomic nervous system are illustrated, along with some of the key features of each division.

The key word above is MOST. Most of the sympathetic system utilizes norepinephrine, but acetylcholine is also found (sweat glands). In addition, the adrenal medulla is considered part of the sympathetic nervous system and it releases epinephrine. Note also that norepinephrine = NE = noradrenaline and that epinephrine = EPI = adrenaline (hence the term *adrenergic*).

SYNTHESIS, STORAGE, RELEASE, AND REMOVAL OF TRANSMITTERS

The synthesis, storage, release, and removal of transmitters is important because there are drugs that target each of these steps.

It is not really necessary to memorize the complete synthesis of each and every neurotransmitter. However, there are a few points that are important. Since it's easier, let's start with acetylcholine.

Acetylcholine is synthesized from acetylCoA and choline. It's action is terminated by acetylcholinesterase.

This is really easy to remember from the names. AcetylCoA plus choline gives you acetylcholine. The "esterase" enzyme breaks down the acetylcholine.

Okay. Now on to norepinephrine and it's friend and relative epinephrine. The synthesis of these two compounds is important to know, at least by name (Fig. 6-3). You might also try to remember the details of the biochemistry if you have time.

The rate-limiting step in the synthesis of norepinephrine and epinephrine is the conversion of tyrosine to DOPA by tyrosine β-hydroxylase. This is not that important pharmacologically, but seems to appear as an exam question in rather unpredictable places.

The effect of norepinephrine is terminated predominantly by reuptake into the neuron from which it was released.

Norepinephrine can also be inactivated by enzymes in the liver (mostly) and brain (some). The degradative enzymes are affectionately called COMT

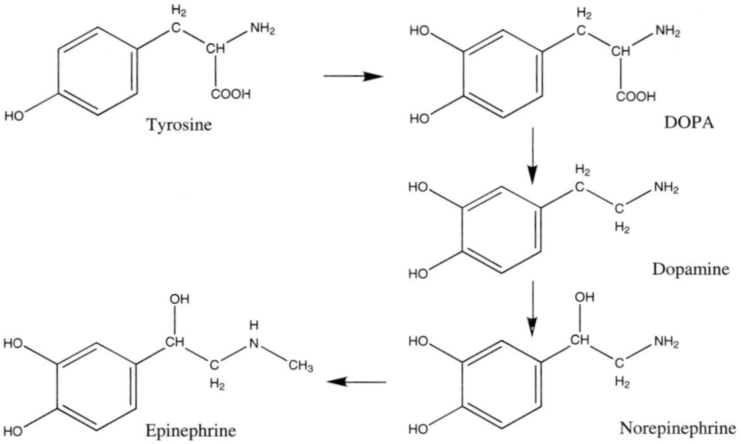

Figure 6-3
The synthesis of norepinephrine and epinephrine are illustrated. Note the close relationship between dopamine, norepinephrine, and epinephrine.

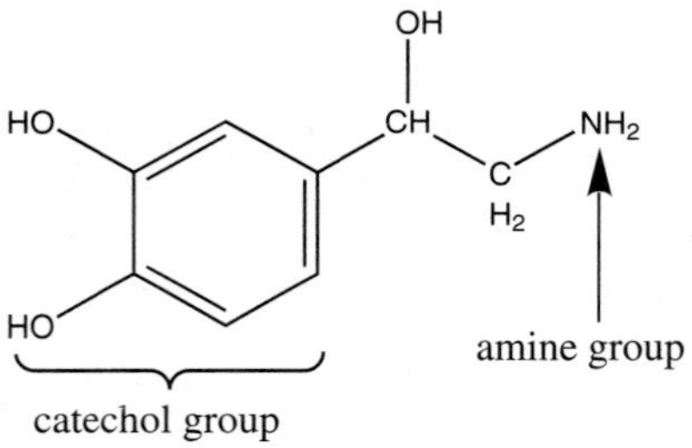

Figure 6-4
The general catecholamine structure is illustrated. The catechol group consists of a benzene ring with two hydroxyl groups.

(catechol-*o*-methyltransferase) and MAO (monoamine oxidase). MAO comes in two forms: A and B.

Note: You will often hear the term *catecholamine*. This refers to the structure of this group of compounds. They have a catechol group and an amine group as shown in Fig. 6-4.

RECEPTORS

At this point, you probably know that there are classes of receptors for neurotransmitters. Each class is now broken down into subtypes. For the BIG PICTURE, do not worry about the subtypes for now.

For simplicity's sake, let's first consider the receptors for acetylcholine.

Receptors for acetylcholine

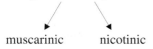

muscarinic   nicotinic

Figure 6-5
The types of acetylcholine receptors are illustrated.

There are two major classes of receptors for acetylcholine: muscarinic and nicotinic (Fig. 6-5).

There are subtypes of muscarinic receptors (M_1, M_2, etc.) and there are at least two types of nicotinic receptors. Do not attempt to memorize these subtypes until you understand the bigger picture.

All of the parasympathetic postganglionic fibers release acetylcholine. At the target organ the acetylcholine interacts with muscarinic receptors.

This should look familiar, since it is the same box that we used before. These muscarinic receptors are predominantly in the viscera (GI tract).

Nicotinic receptors are found at the motor end-plate, in *all* autonomic ganglia and in the adrenal medulla.

Remember the somatic nervous system that controls movement. It utilizes acetylcholine and the receptors are *all* nicotinic. Remember the autonomic ganglia that are present for both the sympathetic and parasympathetic branches. *All* the preganglionic fibers release acetylcholine that interacts with nicotinic receptors. Simply add to this that the adrenal medulla contains nicotinic receptors and you have it made.

Now on to the receptors for norepinephrine. These are more difficult and confusing for students.

Receptors for norepinephrine are divided into α and β receptors. Each of these is then subdivided into α_1 and α_2, and β_1 and β_2.

Receptors for norepinephrine

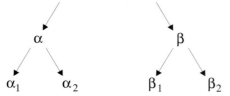

Figure 6-6
The subtypes of receptors for
norepinephrine are illustrated.

There are other α and β receptors, but focus on these four for now (Fig. 6-6). These receptors are found in particular target organs. For example, the heart contains β_1 receptors, while β_2 receptors are found in skeletal muscle blood vessels and the bronchial smooth muscle. This localization of receptor type is the basis of drug therapy. In order to target drug action to the correct organ, drugs have been found (or designed) that primarily affect only one or two receptor types. This is a very important principle of pharmacology and drug therapy.

GENERAL RULES OF INNERVATION

> Many organs are innervated by both the sympathetic and parasympathetic nervous systems. Most of the time the two systems have opposing effects.

When the sympathetic and parasympathetic nervous systems both innervate the same organ system, they tend to have opposite actions. When considering the actions remember that the sympathetic system (no matter which receptor type is involved) is mediating the fight-or-flight response. For example, both the sympathetic and parasympathetic system innervate the heart. The sympathetic system increases heart rate and contractility (in order to run faster), while the parasympathetic system decreases heart rate and contractility (in order to conserve energy). The one exception to the opposite effect rule is on salivary glands. Both the sympathetic and parasympathetic systems increase secretion.

> Important organs that receive innervation from *both* the sympathetic and parasympathetic nervous systems include: heart, eye, bronchial smooth muscle, GI tract smooth muscle, and genitourinary tract smooth muscle.

In the box above, note the absence from the list of the smooth muscles throughout the vascular system (in the arteries).

In the resting state (not in fight-or-flight situations) most dually inner-vated organs are controlled by the parasympathetic system.

This "state dependence" is important when considering drug action. At rest, a drug that blocks the effects of norepinephrine (sympathetic) will have little effect, while a drug that blocks the effects of acetylcholine at muscarinic receptors (parasympathetic) will have a powerful effect. In contrast, in a situation that is dominated by a fight-or-flight response (such as acute trauma or high-stress situation) the blocker of norepinephrine will have a greater effect.

Most books will have a large table of target organs and the effect of activation of the sympathetic versus the parasympathetic nervous system. Look through the table and first rationalize the sympathetic responses to the fight-or-flight response. The pupils should dilate, the heart rate and contractility should increase, the bronchials should dilate, the GI tract should shut down (relax the walls and contract the sphincters), the bladder should shut down (the walls relax and the sphincter contracts), blood should be shunted from the GI tract and skin to the muscles, and metabolism should increase the supply of glucose. This stuff "makes sense" and doesn't need to be memorized.

Most of the vascular smooth muscle is innervated solely by the sympathetic nervous system. This means that blood pressure and peripheral resistance are controlled by the sympathetic nervous system.

Remember that the vascular smooth muscle is the prime example of a target organ that does not have dual innervation.

Contraction of the radial muscle (sympathetic innervation) causes dilation, or mydriasis (expected sympathetic response), while contraction of the circular muscle (parasympathetic innervation) causes constriction or miosis (expected parasympathetic response).

The eye responses can trip up students. Remember *rad*ial muscle causes *d*ilation (my*d*riasis) and the *c*ircular muscle causes *c*onstriction (mi*o*sis) (or no "d" 's in any of those words relating to constriction). On your next visit to the eye doctor, if he or she dilates your pupils, ask what is in the drops.

The heart is the main site for β_1 receptors.

If a drug is specific for β_1 receptors, its main effect will be on the heart. β_1 receptors are also involved in the release of renin from the kidney.

Activation of β_2 receptors relaxes smooth muscle.

This is somewhat a generality, but is useful to help organize your learning. The smooth muscles that contain the β_2 receptors are found in the blood vessels in skeletal muscles (leading to vasodilation), the GI tract, the bronchial walls, the bladder wall, and the pregnant uterus.

Activation of α receptors causes contraction or constriction. Activation of α_1 receptors leads to vasoconstriction.

Again, this is a simplification, but useful to organize your learning. Activation of α receptors contracts blood vessels in the GI tract, contracts the radial muscle in the eye, contracts sphincters in various places, and mediates ejaculation. That last one is the only effect of the sympathetic nervous system that does not fit neatly into our fight-or-flight response.

CHOLINERGIC AGONISTS

·

Organization of Class

Direct Cholinergic Agonists

Cholinesterase Inhibitors

·   ·   ·   ·   ·   ·   ·   ·   ·   ·   ·   ·

ORGANIZATION OF CLASS

Although I have titled this chapter "Cholinergic Agonists," this chapter considers all the drugs that increase activity in cholinergic neurons, sometimes called *cholinomimetics* (because they mimic the action of acetylcholine). There are two main targets of drug action: the postsynaptic receptor and the acetylcholinesterase enzyme that breaks down acetylcholine.

> Direct-acting cholinergic agonists have a direct action on the receptor for acetylcholine. Some drugs are specific for the muscarinic receptor and some are specific for the nicotinic receptor.

First, remind yourself where nicotinic and muscarinic receptors are found.

1. *All* autonomic ganglia have nicotinic receptors.
2. *All* target organs of the parasympathetic nervous system have muscarinic receptors.
3. *All* receptors at the neuromuscular junction are nicotinic receptors.

There are other cholinergic receptors, such as in the central nervous system and in sweat glands innervated by the sympathetic nervous system. Concentrate on the three listed above—add the others later.

The indirect-acting cholinomimetics act by blocking the metabolism of acetylcholine by cholinesterases. These drugs effectively increase the concentration of acetylcholine at *all* cholinergic synapses.

The enzyme that is specific for acetylcholine is called *acetylcholinesterase* and it is found on both the pre- and postsynaptic membranes. There are other cholinesterases that will metabolize acetylcholine and drugs with related structures. These other cholinesterases are sometimes called *pseudocholinesterases* or *nonspecific cholinesterases,* and they are abundant in the liver.

The structure and biochemistry of acetylcholinesterase is well studied and an interesting story. Details can be found in most textbooks.

All cholinomimetics cause the following effects mediated by muscarinic receptors.

Eye: Miosis (constriction of pupil)
CV: Decrease in heart rate and contractility
Resp: Bronchial constriction and increased secretions
GI: Increased motility, relaxation of sphincters
GU: Relaxation of sphincters and bladder wall contraction
Glands: Increased secretion

Basically all of these effects can be predicted based on your knowledge of the effects of the parasympathetic nervous system. Therefore, this is a review and not a list of new things to learn. (We are trying to keep this stuff simple).

> Cholinomimetics will also cause effects at the neuromuscular junction, if they affect nicotinic receptors. This includes all of the indirect-acting agents.

We will come back to the effects of drugs at the neuromuscular junction later.

DIRECT CHOLINERGIC AGONISTS

ESTERS	ALKALOIDS
BETHANECHOL	muscarine
methacholine	pilocarpine
carbachol	arecoline

These drugs are traditionally divided into two groups: esters of choline that are structurally related to acetylcholine (-*chol.* in name) and the alkaloids that are not related to acetylcholine and are generally plant derivatives. The *only* reason that this distinction is important is that the alkaloids, because of their complex structure, are not metabolized by cholinesterases.

> The effects of *all* of these agents are exclusively muscarinic.

That is a very sweeping statement that is not entirely true. However, the therapeutically useful drugs in reasonable concentrations are muscarinic. The effects of these drugs are listed above, but also can be deduced from your knowledge of the parasympathetic nervous system. The differences between the drugs are related to their resistance to cholinesterase activity and specificity for nicotinic receptors.

> BETHANECHOL is used in the treatment of urinary retention.

Of the drugs in the group, bethanechol is the most clinically useful. It is used to treat urinary retention in the postoperative period and in a neurogenic bladder.

The side effects of these drugs are directly related to their interaction with muscarinic receptors.

If you know the actions of these drugs, you also know the side effects. That means no new lists to memorize. Side effects are often listed as sweating (increased secretion), salivation, GI distress, and cramps (due to increased motility).

See how easy this is to learn!

Nicotine is a direct agonist at nicotinic receptors.

Nicotine is used therapeutically for helping patients stop smoking.

CHOLINESTERASE INHIBITORS

These drugs are also often divided into two or three groups based on their structure. Words like mono-quaternary amine, bis-quaternary amine, carbamate, and organophosphate appear in books. For our purposes, we will divide the drugs into two groups.

REVERSIBLE INHIBITORS	IRREVERSIBLE INHIBITORS ORGANOPHOSPHATES
Water Soluble	*Lipid Soluble/Cross the BBB*
ambenonium	isoflurophate
demecarium	echothiophate
EDROPHONIUM	diisopropyl flurophosphate
NEOSTIGMINE	parathion
physostigmine	malathion
PYRIDOSTIGMINE	soman
	sarin

The reversible inhibitors include the quaternary amines and the carbamates and are the clinically useful drugs. They compete with acetylcholine for the active site on the cholinesterase enzyme. They include the -*stigmines* and the -*niums*. The irreversible inhibitors phosphorylate the enzyme and inactivate it. These cholinesterase inhibitors are widely used as insecticides and are "nerve gases." Because the organophosphates are lipid soluble they rapidly cross all membranes, including skin and the blood–brain barrier (BBB). The organophosphates include the -*phates* and the -*thions*.

These drugs have all the same actions (and side effects) as the direct-acting drugs (muscarinic). In addition, they have effects at the neuromuscular junction (nicotinic).

These drugs will cause the same side effects as the direct cholinergic agonists. There is nothing new here.

These drugs also effect nicotinic receptors, primarily at the neuromuscular junction. This is the basis of their therapeutic use. They cause fasciculations and weakness in normal people and can improve muscle strength in patients with myasthenia gravis. Myasthenia gravis is an immune disease in which there is a loss of acetylcholine receptors at the neuromuscular junction.

These drugs can have effects on the cholinergic system in the central nervous system, if the drug can cross the blood–brain barrier. The effects range from tremor, anxiety, and restlessness, to coma. The organophosphates, because of their lipid solubility, rapidly cross into the central nervous system.

EDROPHONIUM is used in the diagnosis of myasthenia gravis.

Edrophonium is a short-acting cholinesterase inhibitor that is administered IV to patients suspected of having weakness due to myasthenia gravis. If they have myasthenia, then the drug will dramatically improve muscle strength. If they do not have myasthenia gravis, can you think of the effects of administration of a cholinesterase inhibitor?*

*How about increased secretions and GI cramping (due to increased motility)

NEOSTIGMINE and PYRIDOSTIGMINE are used in the treatment of myasthenia gravis.

These drugs act in the same way as edrophonium, but are longer
acting. Therefore, they are used for treatment and not for diagnosis.

Other uses of the reversible cholinesterase inhibitors are in the treatment of open-angle glaucoma and the reversal of nondepolarizing
neuromuscular blockade after surgery.

A number of the drugs are listed for these uses. If you have the energy
you can memorize some.

There are no therapeutic uses for the irreversible cholinesterase inhibitors.

These agents are of interest because of the pharmacology involved (of
course, I'm biased) and because of poisoning.

PRALIDOXIME and ATROPINE are used to treat poisoning with
organophosphates.

The organophosphates phosphorylate the cholinesterase enzyme, thus
inactivating it. Pralidoxime is able to hydrolyze the phosphate bond and
reactivate the enzyme. This works well if the enzyme–phosphate complex
has not "aged" (a story too complex for this book, but quite interesting).
Also, pralidoxime does not cross the blood–brain barrier, so it is not effective in reversing the central nervous system effects of the organophosphate.
Atropine (muscarinic antagonist) can also be used in the treatment of
organophosphate poisoning because it will block the effects of the excess
acetylcholine, but only at the muscarinic receptors. It has no effect at the
neuromuscular junction (nicotinic).

CHOLINERGIC ANTAGONISTS

·

Organization of Class

Muscarinic Antagonists

Ganglionic Blockers

Neuromuscular Blockers

·   ·   ·   ·   ·   ·   ·   ·   ·   ·   ·   ·

ORGANIZATION OF CLASS

This group of drugs antagonize the effects of acetylcholine. Most of the drugs are antagonists directly at the nicotinic or muscarinic receptor. Some of the agents act on the ion channel that is associated with the nicotinic receptor and still others block acetylcholine release.

MUSCARINIC ANTAGONISTS

The prototypic muscarinic antagonist is ATROPINE.

In this group of compounds it is useful to consider a prototype drug and then compare the other drugs to it. The prototype drug here is atropine.

All of the muscarinic antagonists are competitive antagonists of the binding of acetylcholine to the muscarinic receptor.

These drugs compete with acetylcholine for binding to the muscarinic receptor. They have no intrinsic activity. In other words, in the absence of acetylcholine they would have no effect.

The effects and side effects of these drugs are the opposite of the drugs (the cholinomimetics) considered in the last chapter.

Eye: Mydriasis, cycloplegia (blurred vision)
Skin: Reduced sweating, flushing
GI: Reduced motility and secretions
CV: Decreased heart rate (low doses), increased heart rate (high doses)
Respiratory: Bronchial dilation and decreased secretion
GU: Urinary retention
CNS: Drowsiness, hallucinations, coma

Compare these effects to those listed in the previous chapter. The important ones to remember are the common side effects of drugs that have anticholinergic properties (many of the CNS drugs), that is, dry eyes, dry mouth, blurred vision, constipation, and urinary retention. If you master the anticholinergic effects now, it will save you considerable effort later.

There are many muscarinic antagonists currently available and their names do not all sound alike. Some name recognition exercises may be useful here.

ATROPINE	trihexylphenidyl	SCOPOLAMINE
benztropine	dicyclomine	glycopyrrolate
cyclopentolate	IPRATROPIUM	tropicamide
propantheline	oxybutynin	pirenzepine

Some of these drugs have particular uses. These names should be learned first and then the others added later.

ATROPINE and SCOPOLAMINE are used preoperatively to reduce secretions.

SCOPOLAMINE is used to prevent motion sickness.

IPRATROPIUM is used in the treatment of chronic obstructive pulmonary disease (COPD) to produce bronchodilation.

Other of the drugs are used to inhibit involuntary bladder contractions, to produce mydriasis, to treat Parkinson's disease, and as adjuncts in the treatment of irritable bowel syndrome.

GANGLIONIC BLOCKERS

Ganglionic blockers work by interfering with the postsynaptic action of acetylcholine. They block the action of acetylcholine at the nicotinic receptor of all autonomic ganglia. Drugs have not yet been developed that can distinguish the sympathetic and parasympathetic ganglia. The nicotinic receptors in autonomic ganglia differ slightly from nicotinic receptors at the neuromuscular junction. Drugs have been developed that have selectivity for each type of nicotinic receptor.

Only three drugs are commonly listed in textbooks in this drug class and only one has a particular use to remember.

hexamethonium
trimethaphan
mecamylamine

Hexamethonium is often listed in books as the prototype drug, but it is old and out-of-date. You should probably recognize the name.

> Trimethaphan is used to produce controlled hypotension in certain surgical procedures and in the emergency treatment of hypertension.

NEUROMUSCULAR BLOCKERS

These drugs are a little out-of-place in the section on autonomics. However, since they interact with nicotinic receptors we will consider them here. It actually makes some of the thinking and learning about the drugs and their side effects easier. And we are definitely for making things easier!

Drugs that competitively bind to the nicotinic receptor are used as neuromuscular blockers. The drugs are classified as depolarizing or non-depolarizing blockers based on their mechanism of action. Isn't it great when the drug group is named by its mechanism? The depolarizing agent binds to the receptor, opens the ion channel, depolarizes the end-plate, and then gets stuck. Therefore, it is called a depolarizing blocker. The nondepolarizing blockers bind to the receptor, but do not open the ion channel.

All of these drugs bind to all nicotinic receptors (neuromuscular junction and autonomic ganglia) and some actually bind muscarinic receptors to a small extent. The neuromuscular blockers act relatively selectively at the nicotinic receptor at the neuromuscular junction. They vary in their potency in each area and in their duration of action.

> The competitive neuromuscular blocking drugs are used to produce skeletal muscle relaxation.

Think for a moment!! Why did I specify skeletal muscle? How do you relax smooth muscle? (Hint: the smooth muscle is controlled by the autonomic nervous system).

To make things simpler there is only one depolarizing agent that you need to know.

> SUCCINYLCHOLINE is a depolarizing neuromuscular blocker.

Succinylcholine will depolarize the neuromuscular junction. It has a brief action. It's use has been associated with malignant hyperthermia, which can be FATAL.

Now, on to the nondepolarizing blockers. There are a number of these.

NONDEPOLARIZING BLOCKERS		
d-TUBOCURARINE	mivacurium	pancuronium
pipecuronium	vecuronium	doxacurium
atracurium	rocurium	GALLAMINE
metocurine iodide		

Notice that all of the names contain -cur-, except gallamine. This should make it easier to recognize the names when you see them. Gallamine and *d*-tubocurarine seem to appear most often on exams, so learn these names first.

The neuromuscular junction (and other cholinergic synapses) can be blocked by drugs that block the release of acetylcholine.

Botulinum toxin blocks the release of acetylcholine at all cholinergic synapses.

Normally, we think of botulinum toxin as a very potent poison that causes botulism. Recently, it has found a therapeutic use treating prolonged muscle spasm. A small amount of the toxin is injected directly into the muscle fiber to cause that muscle to relax.

DANTROLENE is used to treat malignant hyperthermia.

That was a short aside. There was no good place to put dantrolene and you need to know its name and use. You may also wish to learn its mechanism of action.

ADRENERGIC AGONISTS
·

Organization of Class

Direct-Acting Agonists

Dopamine

Indirect-Acting Agents

Cardiovascular Effects of Norepinephrine, Epinephrine, and Isoproterenol

·   ·   ·   ·   ·   ·   ·   ·   ·   ·   ·   ·

ORGANIZATION OF CLASS

This chapter considers the drugs that mimic the effects of adrenergic nerve stimulation (or stimulation of the adrenal medulla). In other words, these compounds mimic the effects of norepinephrine or epinephrine. Remember that the actions of the sympathetic nervous system are mediated through α and β receptors. These drugs are sometimes referred to as *adrenomimetics* or *sympathomimetics*.

Reminder:

$\alpha_1 =$ most vascular smooth muscle: agonists contract
$\beta_1 =$ heart: agonists increase rate
$\beta_2 =$ respiratory and uterine smooth muscle: agonists relax

There are other effects of sympathetic stimulation, but the three listed in the box are the most important.

Suppose that you have a patient, a 65-year-old male with a long history of reactive airway disease. He recently had a mild heart attack. Now he comes to you with a flare-up of his airway disease. You want to relax the smooth muscle of the bronchials without stimulating the heart (you don't want to jeopardize his heart by increasing the work load). If you could stimulate the β_2 receptors in the respiratory tract specifically, then you could successfully treat your patient. This is why it is important to know where the receptors are located and which drugs are specific for which receptors.

The drugs are often divided into direct and indirect-acting drugs. This is a useful distinction for a number of reasons. The indirect-acting drugs do not bind to specific receptors, but act by releasing stored norepinephrine. This means that their actions are nonspecific. The direct-acting drugs bind to the receptors, so specificity of action is a possibility.

The drugs are also sometimes divided into catecholamines and noncatecholamines. This is yet another division based on structures (and we do not focus on structures). This distinction is useful for one concept. Remember that norepinephrine is metabolized by COMT and MAO? Well, the other catecholamines are also metabolized by these enzymes. The noncatecholamines are not.

DIRECT-ACTING AGONISTS

The focus here is to learn the specificity of the drugs for the receptor targets. If you know the effect of stimulation of the target receptors, then you can deduce the drug actions and adverse effects. A drug could activate only α receptors, only β receptors, or both types of receptors.

Only EPINEPHRINE and NOREPINEPHRINE activate both α and β receptors.

This is an oversimplification, but a useful starting point. The rest of the direct-acting drugs act on *either* α or β receptors (Fig. 9-1). Epinephrine has approximately equal effects at α and β receptors. In addition, it has approximately equal effects at β_1 and β_2 receptors. Epinephrine has a number of uses, including the treatment of allergic reactions, the treatment of shock, to control localized bleeding, and to prolong the action of local anesthetics.

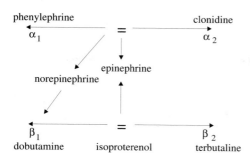

Figure 9-1

A classification of adrenergic agonists is presented. Affinity for the α receptors is shown on the top and affinity for the β receptors is shown on the bottom. Epinephrine and norepinephrine have affinity for both α and β receptors and are, therefore, placed in the middle.

NOREPINEPHRINE has a relatively low affinity for β_2 receptors.

Norepinephrine activates both α and β receptors, but activates β_1 receptors more than β_2 receptors. Because of the relatively low affinity for β_2 receptors, norepinephrine is not as useful in the treatment of bronchospasm as epinephrine. Why? Because the smooth muscle of the bronchioles is relaxed by the activation of β_2 receptors.

Let us now move on to consider the α- and β-specific drugs. The α-specific drugs are easier, so let's start there.

DRUG	RECEPTOR EFFECT	CLINICAL EFFECT
PHENYLEPHRINE	α_1 Agonist	Nasal decongestant
CLONIDINE	α_2 Agonist	Decreases blood pressure through a central action

The main effect of α_1 stimulation (with an agonist such as phenylephrine) is vasoconstriction. Local application of a vasoconstrictor to the nasal passages will decrease blood flow locally and decrease secretions (i.e., nasal decongestant). The action of clonidine is more complex and beyond the scope of this chapter. However, it is useful to know that it is a specific α_2 agonist.

DRUG	RECEPTOR EFFECT	CLINICAL EFFECT
DOBUTAMINE	β_1 agonist	Increases heart rate and cardiac output
ISOPROTERENOL	$\beta_1 = \beta_2$ agonist	
TERBUTALINE	β_2 agonist	Relieve
ALBUTEROL		bronchoconstriction
metaproterenol		

Basically, there is a spectrum of drugs that fall on the line from β_1 to β_2 (see Fig. 9-1). Dobutamine is closer to the β_1 end. Terbutaline and its relatives are closer to the β_2 end. Isoproterenol falls in the middle.

DOPAMINE

Dopamine is a catecholamine by structure and is a precursor to norepinephrine (cf. Fig. 6-3). There are also dopamine receptors throughout the body and in the central nervous system. At high doses dopamine acts much like epinephrine.

> At low doses DOPAMINE causes renal and coronary vasodilatation. It also activates β_1 receptors in the heart.

In the treatment of shock, dopamine will increase heart rate and cardiac output, while simultaneously dilating the renal and coronary arteries. The action of dopamine in the renal vascular bed is used to try and preserve renal function.

INDIRECT-ACTING AGENTS

The indirect-acting sympathomimetic agents act by releasing previously stored norepinephrine. Thus, the effects of these drugs are widespread and nonspecific.

> Ephedrine and phenylpropanolamine are nasal decongestants. Phenylpropanolamine has also been used as an appetite suppressant.

If you can't remember these drugs, it is not a great loss. Be careful not to confuse phenylephrine (the specific α_1 agonist) with these two similarly named indirect agents.

AMPHETAMINE, and its relative methylphenidate, are central nervous system stimulants used to treat attention deficit hyperactivity disorder in children.

Amphetamine and others of its relatives are indirect-acting sympathomimetics that have been abused because of their psychostimulant abilities.

CARDIOVASCULAR EFFECTS OF NOREPINEPHRINE, EPINEPHRINE, AND ISOPROTERENOL

Before we leave the adrenergic activators, it is useful to consider in detail the cardiovascular actions of norepinephrine, epinephrine, and isoproterenol. Some books will also consider dopamine. Consider the effects of these agents on heart rate, cardiac output, total peripheral resistance, and mean arterial pressure. If you find these easy enough, then add in systolic and diastolic blood pressure.

Norepinephrine increases total peripheral resistance and mean arterial pressure.

Through stimulation of α receptors, norepinephrine causes constriction of all major vascular beds. This causes an increase in resistance and pressure. Norepinephrine has less effect on the β_1 receptors in the heart, so the effects on heart rate and cardiac output are complex. The increase in blood pressure causes a reflex increase in parasympathetic output to the heart to slow it down. Therefore, heart rate often decreases after administration of norepinephrine.

Epinephrine predominately affects the heart through β_1 receptors, causing an increase in heart rate and cardiac output.

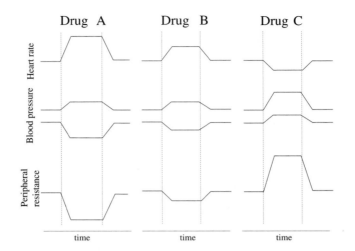

Figure 9-2
The effect of an intravenous infusion of three different agents on heart rate, blood pressure (systolic and diastolic), and peripheral vascular resistance are graphed. The drugs were administered during the time indicated by the vertical dashed lines. Which graph represents the effect of epinephrine? norepinephrine? isoproterenol?

While epinephrine activates all α and β receptors, if given systemically its cardiovascular effects are predominated by effects on the heart. It increases heart rate, stroke volume, and cardiac output. The effects of epinephrine on blood pressure and peripheral resistance are dose-dependent. At low doses, there is a fall in peripheral resistance from vasodilation in the skeletal muscle beds. There is usually an increase in systolic pressure and a decrease in diastolic blood pressure. The mean arterial pressure may increase, decrease, or stay the same.

Isoproterenol causes a marked decrease in total peripheral resistance and an increase in heart rate and cardiac output.

Remember that isoproterenol is β only. Therefore, there is no vasoconstriction of the vascular smooth muscle. The vasodilatation in the skeletal muscle beds (β) is unopposed. This results in a net decrease in peripheral resistance. Isoproterenol also stimulates the β_1 receptor in the heart. This results in a direct stimulation of heart rate and stroke volume.

Which of the graphs in Fig. 9-2 represents the changes due to epinephrine? norepinephrine? isoproterenol?*

*Answers: (A) isoproterenol; (B) epinephrine; (C) norepinephrine

ADRENERGIC ANTAGONISTS

·

Organization of Class

Central Blockers

α-Blockers

β-Blockers

Labetalol

· · · · · · · · · · · ·

ORGANIZATION OF CLASS

The effects of the sympathetic nervous system can be blocked either by decreasing sympathetic outflow from the brain, suppressing release of norepinephrine from terminals, or by blocking postsynaptic receptors. Adrenergic antagonists reduce the effectiveness of sympathetic nerve stimulation and the effects of exogenously applied agonists, such as isoproterenol. Most often the receptor antagonists are divided into α-receptor antagonists and β-receptor antagonists. This will work for us also.

CENTRAL BLOCKERS

Here we finally get to a short discussion of α_2-receptor agonists. Yes, I did write agonists, not antagonists—and in a chapter on antagonists!!

α_2 Agonists reduce sympathetic nerve activity and are used to treat hypertension.

α_2-Receptor activation inhibits the sympathetic output from the brain and inhibits release of norepinephrine from nerve terminals. We have already listed one—clonidine. There are at least two more: guanabenz and guanfacine. α-Methyl-DOPA is metabolized to α-methylnorepinephrine, which is also an α_2 agonist. Because they reduce the output from the brain to the sympathetic nervous system, the α_2 agonists have found usefulness and purpose in life in the treatment of hypertension.

α-BLOCKERS

There are a large number of compounds that possess some α-blocking activity in addition to some primary action. For example, the antipsychotics have α-antagonist properties. In the case of the antipsychotics, these actions are considered side effects. The drugs that we will consider here have their primary action as α antagonists.

Most of the α antagonists allow vasodilation and, thus, decrease blood pressure.

Remember that α-activation results in vasoconstriction. It should follow that α-blockade will produce vasodilation. This is particularly true when the sympathetic nervous system is firing. For example, the sympathetic nervous system is more active in maintaining blood pressure when you are standing than when you are lying down. This is why α-blockade results in a greater decrease in blood pressure in the standing position. This is called *postural hypotension.*

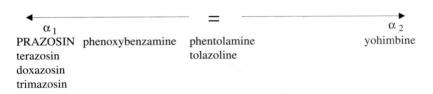

Figure 10-1
The relative affinities of various antagonists for the α receptor are schematized.

> The side effects of the α-blockers are directly related to their α-blocking activity.

For the most part, the side effects of the α-blockers are intuitive. The most common are postural hypotension and reflex tachycardia.

Of course, you remember that there are subtypes of the α receptors. You could probably have guessed that there are drugs that are specific antagonists at the α_1 receptor and others that are specific for the α_2 receptor (Fig. 10-1). Phentolamine and tolazoline are about equal in effectiveness at α_1 and α_2 receptors, phenoxybenzamine moves down the line towards α_1. The rest of the drugs are selective for α_1. Notice that this later group all ends in *-azosin.*

All of the α-blockers are reversible inhibitors of the α receptor, except phenoxybenzamine, which is irreversible.

> The *-azosins,* such as PRAZOSIN, are used in the treatment of hypertension.

Because of their specificity for α_1 receptors, prazosin and its relatives (terazosin, doxazosin, and trimazosin) have fewer side effects.

> Yohimbine is a selective antagonist at α_2 receptors. It has no clinical role.

If you can't remember that one, don't worry.

β-BLOCKERS

First, remind yourself of the localization and action of the β receptors. β_1 receptors are found in the heart, and activation leads to an increase in heart rate and contractility. β_2 receptors are found in the smooth muscle of the respiratory tract, uterus, and blood vessels. Activation leads to relaxation of the smooth muscle.

$\beta_1 =$ heart: antagonism leads to a decrease in heart rate.

$\beta_2 =$ smooth muscle: antagonism leads to contraction of the smooth muscle. This translates into bronchial constriction, which may be dangerous in asthmatics.

The actions of β-blockers on blood pressure are complex. Remember that α receptors control most of the vascular smooth muscle in an unopposed fashion. Chronic administration of β-blockers will, however, decrease blood pressure.

The β-blockers have widespread use in the management of cardiac arrhythmias, angina, and hypertension.

β-blockers are also used in the treatment of hyperthyroidism, glaucoma, migraines, and anxiety.

β-blockers should be used with caution in diabetics.

Recall that the metabolic effects of sympathetic stimulation (glycogenolysis, gluconeogenesis, lipolysis) are mediated by β receptors. In response to hypoglycemia (low sugar), the sympathetic nervous system stimulates an increase in blood sugar through β receptors. Blocking this response with a β-blocker will cause the blood sugar to remain low. In addition, the reflex increase in heart rate that occurs in response to hypoglycemia is also blocked by β-blockers. Many diabetics can detect a drop in blood sugar by the reflex increase in heart rate. If you are giving them β-blockers, they lose this early warning sign.

Since the major use of these drugs is for cardiac reasons, β_1-selective antagonists are often referred to as *cardioselective.*

Because the β-receptors in the heart are β_1, drugs that are selective for the β_1 receptor are referred to as *cardioselective.*

NON-CARDIOSELECTIVE	CARDIOSELECTIVE
PROPRANOLOL	acebutolol
carteolol	atenolol
levobunolol	betaxolol
nadolol	bisoprolol
penbutolol	esmolol
pindolol	metoprolol
timolol	

Using the names only, there is no good way to distinguish the cardio-selective ones from the others. On the bright side, every student can recognize the *-olol* of the β-blockers. There is a tendency for the cardioselective ones to be closer to the beginning of the alphabet than the nonselective ones.

Besides their cardioselectivity, these drugs vary in duration of action and metabolism.

The adverse effects of these drugs are, for the most part, directly related to their β-blocking abilities.

The drugs can cause bronchoconstriction and decreased heart rate and cardiac output. Any of these actions could be considered side effects.

LABETALOL

First, notice that labetalol does not end in *-olol,* but in *-alol.* Use this to remember that labetalol is different from the other β-blockers.

Labetalol has both α- and β-blocking activity.

Because of the ratio of β-to-α activity, labetalol is most often listed as a β-blocker with some α-blocking activity. It is nonselective at the β receptor, but is specific for α_1 receptors. Its effects are kind of complex, but make interesting reading. You can use it to test your understanding of the adrenergic receptors and their actions.

DRUGS THAT AFFECT THE CARDIOVASCULAR SYSTEM

·

DRUGS USED TO TREAT HEART FAILURE

·

Organization of Class

Inotropic Agents

Angiotensin-Converting Enzyme Inhibitors

Dobutamine and Dopamine

Vasodilators

· · · · · · · · · · · · ·

ORGANIZATION OF CLASS

Heart failure occurs when the heart can no longer pump enough blood to meet the demands of the body.

> Treatment of heart failure is targeted toward increasing contractility, decreasing preload, or decreasing afterload.

Treatment of heart failure involves increasing the contractility of the heart, thereby increasing cardiac output. Alternatively, preload or afterload can be reduced. Preload is essentially the amount of blood that fills the ventricle before (pre) the heart pumps. The greater the amount of blood in the ventricle, the harder the heart has to pump to move the blood. Afterload is the pressure in the arteries that the heart has to push against to get the blood out of the ventricle.

The most useful organization of this group of drugs is by mechanism of action. There are really only a few new drugs here, so don't worry too much. It may be more helpful to spend a few minutes at this point reviewing some cardiac physiology.

INOTROPIC AGENTS

Inotropic agents increase the contractility of the heart. Therefore, they improve heart failure by increasing cardiac output.

CARDIAC GLYCOSIDES

The cardiac glycosides were originally isolated from the *Digitalis* plant. Hence the names digitalis, digoxin, and digitoxin. The term digitalis is a general term that usually means digoxin.

The cardiac glycosides (DIGOXIN and DIGITOXIN) improve myocardial contractility. They inhibit the Na^+,K^+-ATPase.

These drugs will inhibit the sodium–potassium ATPase and enhance the release of intracellular calcium from the sarcoplasmic reticulum. This increase in intracellular calcium causes an increase in the force of contraction of the myocytes throughout the heart. In addition to their general use in heart failure, both digoxin and digitoxin will slow the ventricular rate in atrial flutter or fibrillation by increasing the sensitivity of the AV node to vagal stimulation. This makes them antiarrhythmic drugs also (see Chap. 13).

Somehow, someway, questions always appear comparing digoxin and digitoxin, so be forewarned and prepared.

1. Notice that the word digitoxin is *longer* (*more* letters) than digoxin.

Digitoxin has a *longer* half life and has *more* metabolites and is *more* absorbed from the GI tract and is *more* protein bound than digoxin.

---

2. Conversely, digoxin is a *shorter* word (*fewer* letters) than digitoxin.

Digoxin has a *shorter* half-life, no (the ultimate *less*) metabolites, is *less* absorbed from the GI tract, and is *less* protein bound.

That said, digoxin is more commonly used than digitoxin.

The cardiac glycosides have a low therapeutic index.

The therapeutic index is the LD_{50} over the ED_{50}. A low therapeutic index means that the plasma concentration that causes serious toxicity (may be FATAL) is only slightly higher than the therapeutic dose. The therapeutic index is between 1.6 and 2.5 for the cardiac glycosides. The toxicity of the cardiac glycosides is affected by the serum potassium level. Therefore, toxicity is more common in patients receiving potassium-wasting diuretics, who have low serum potassium levels. This is quite important, since many patients with heart failure are on "dig. and diuretics" (digoxin and a diuretic).

Toxicity due to cardiac glycosides can be manifested by:
  Arrhythmias
  Anorexia, nausea, and diarrhea
  Drowsiness and fatigue
  Visual disturbances

It is the arrhythmias that can be life-threatening.

PHOSPHODIESTERASE INHIBITORS

Some books will list amrinone and milrinone as antiarrhythmic drugs used to treat heart failure. Other books classify them by their structure—bipyridines. I find this kind of confusing, so I will just group them by their presumed mechanism of action. Milrinone is a newer version of amrinone. It is more potent, but otherwise similar.

> Amrinone inhibits phosphodiesterase (PDE). It increases contractility, stroke volume, ejection fraction, and heart rate.

Since phosphodiesterase is the enzyme that breaks open cAMP, phosphodiesterase inhibitors increase levels of cAMP. Inhibition of a particular isoform of phosphodiesterase (PDE III) is associated with increased myocardial contractility. An increase in cAMP in smooth muscle leads to inhibition of contraction. Thus, phosphodiesterase inhibitors will also cause vasodilatation. Amrinone is only administered intravenously, so is only useful for short-term management. A new phosphodiesterase inhibitor is now available—flosequin. (Too bad it has such an odd name!)

ANGIOTENSIN-CONVERTING ENZYME INHIBITORS

There is a very important enzyme in the renin–angiotensin system that you should have heard about by now. It is called peptidyl-dipeptide hydrolase, peptidyl-dipeptidase, or (most commonly) angiotensin-converting enzyme (ACE). This enzyme converts angiotensin I to angiotensin II, which is a potent vasoconstricting substance.

> Angiotensin-converting enzyme (ACE) inhibitors block the synthesis of angiotensin II.

Blocking the synthesis of angiotensin II leads to a decrease in levels of this circulating vasoconstrictor, which results in a decrease in blood pressure (i.e., afterload). ACE inhibitors also reduce aldosterone secretion, which results in a net water loss. This adds to the decrease in afterload. The decrease in afterload is the desired effect for the treatment of heart failure.

The currently available ACE inhibitors are listed in the table below. There may be newer ones available by the time you read this chapter. Feel free to add to the table as needed.

CAPTOPRIL	benazepril
lisinopril	fosinopril
pentapril	quinapril
ramipril	ENALAPRIL

ACE inhibitors have found a number of uses, most prominently in the treatment of hypertension (see Chap. 14) and heart failure. In response to the decrease in blood pressure there is no reflex increase in heart rate, cardiac output, or contractility. These agents lack metabolic side effects.

DOBUTAMINE AND DOPAMINE

This is just a reminder from the autonomics section.

DOBUTAMINE is a β_1 agonist. At moderate doses it increases contractility of the heart without changing blood pressure or heart rate.

Dobutamine is used to increase cardiac output in heart failure and can be used in the treatment of shock. Dobutamine has some α^1 and β_2 agonist effects that play a role in maintaining peripheral vascular resistance. It is only given intravenously, so its use is limited.

DOPAMINE has dopamine receptor agonist activity and, like dobutamine, is used in the acute treatment of heart failure.

In patients with impaired renal function, the use of dopamine (instead of dobutamine) may preserve renal blood flow and, as a result, renal function.

VASODILATORS

Dilation of the venous side of things will reduce preload. Dilation of the arterial side will reduce afterload. Both of these actions will improve symptoms in a patient with heart failure, even though there is no direct action on the heart. The vasodilators are covered in detail in the antihypertensives chapter (Chap. 14).

ANTIANGINAL AGENTS

·

Organization of Class

Nitrates

Calcium Channel Blockers

β-Blockers

· · · · · · · · · · · ·

ORGANIZATION OF CLASS

Angina (chest pain) is a warning sign that the heart is not getting enough oxygen for its work load. Usually this means that blood flow to the heart is reduced. The treatment strategies include increasing blood flow to the heart with angioplasty (mechanically dilating the coronary artery) or bypass surgery. Pharmacologically, angina is treated by reducing the work load of the heart or by increasing blood flow in the coronary vessels. The goal of either approach is to equalize the supply and demand of oxygen to the heart (reminds me of economics class).

So, let's divide the drugs according to their mechanism of action. We can use nitrates or calcium channel blockers for their vasodilating effects. This will decrease the work load of the heart by decreasing preload (volume filling ventricle) or afterload (pressure heart pumps against). The vasodilators maymay also have a direct effect on the coronary arteries. If the coronary arteries dilate, there is an increase in blood flow (oxygen supply) to the heart. Use of β-blockers will slow the heart rate. This will decrease the work load of the heart also.

VASODILATORS	
Nitrates	*Calcium Channel Blockers*
NITROGLYCERIN	VERAPAMIL
isosorbide dinitrate	DILTIAZEM
isosorbide mononitrate	NIFEDIPINE
amyl nitrate	nicardipine
	isradipine
	nimodipine
	bepridil
	amlodipine
	felodipine

DRUGS THAT SLOW THE HEART
β-Blockers
PROPRANOLOL
nadolol
metoprolol
atenolol

Notice that the nitrates all have nitro or nitrate in the name. This makes them easy to identify. The calcium channel blockers all end in -*dipine, -mil,* or *-dil,* except diltiazem. Don't confuse diltiazem with diazepam (a benzodiazepine used as a sedative, Chap. 18). You may use the *dil* at the beginning of diltiazem to match it with the *-mil* and *-dil* endings, if you are really stuck. There are many more β-blockers than those in this table. Be sure you know which β-blockers your book or class handouts consider useful in the treatment of angina. Feel free to add or delete drugs from the table, as needed.

NITRATES

The nitrates are very effective in the treatment of angina. They dilate blood vessels and reduce cardiac preload.

In spite of their use for many years in the treatment of angina, the mechanism of action of the nitrates is not crystal clear (it is actually kind of muddy). It is now thought that these drugs work by conversion to nitric oxide. The nitric oxide increases intracellular cGMP and this leads to smooth muscle relaxation. At higher concentrations the nitrates decrease afterload. Therefore, the nitrates restore the balance between oxygen demand and oxygen supply by changing the work load of the heart.

NITROGLYCERIN is the most commonly used antianginal agent. It is the DRUG OF CHOICE for relieving acute coronary spasm.

Nitroglycerin is often administered sublingually for rapid onset of action, but can be applied transdermally for a longer duration of action. If taken orally, it is subject to extensive first-pass metabolism in the liver. It's effectivness against coronary spasm suggests a direct vasodilatory effect on the coronary arteries.

Amyl nitrate is also used to treat acute attacks of angina. It is administered by inhalation of the crushed capsule.

Isosorbide dinitrate is used for prophylaxis of angina.

For prevention of anginal attacks, a drug is needed that is orally active and has a relatively long half-life. Nitroglycerin does not meet those qualifications. Isosorbide dinitrate does.

Headaches and postural hypotension are common side effects of the use of nitrates.

These side effects do not need to be memorized. Can you see that they are directly related to the mechanism of action of the nitrates (vasodilatation)? Too much vasodilatation peripherally leads to postural hypotension (the blood vessels cannot contract and maintain blood pressure when you stand up), and dilation of cerebral vessels is thought to lead to headaches.

There is also the interesting story of tolerance to the effects of nitrates. It is too low down on the trivial list to include here, but you should at least note that it occurs.

CALCIUM CHANNEL BLOCKERS

> Calcium channel blockers inhibit the entrance of calcium into cells. They cause a decrease in afterload.

I hope that the above statement sounded simplistic! Isn't it nice when the mechanism of action is the name of the group of drugs? Vascular tone and contraction are largely determined by the availability of extracellular calcium. When the entry of calcium into smooth muscle cells of the arteries is inhibited, the vessel will dilate. In general, arteries are more sensitive to the effects of calcium channel blockers than are veins. The vasodilatation produced by calcium channel blockers leads to a decrease in afterload and a decrease in the work of the heart. This restores the balance of the supply and demand of oxygen by the heart.

There are many calcium channel blockers and the list seems to get longer every year. The agents differ in pharmacokinetic properties, potency, and selectivity of action. More details about the vasodilatory action of the calcium channel blockers are in the chapter on antihypertensives (Chap. 14).

> The most common side effects of the calcium channel blockers are related to the vasodilatation (headaches, dizziness, hypotension, etc.).

Remember that the side effects are a direct extension of their action. That way there is nothing new to memorize. Besides, don't these side effects look a lot like the side effects of the nitrates?

Just a few more trivial facts for those of you that want more!!!

1. Nifedipine is useful in the treatment of variant angina (spasm).
2. Verapamil was the drug of choice for the treatment of paroxysmal supraventricular tachycardia. Now it has to play second fiddle to adenosine.

3. Nimodipine is useful in the treatment of spasm of the cerebral vessels after subarachnoid hemorrhage.

β-BLOCKERS

Since an increase in sympathetic activity is a common feature of anginal attacks and this results in an increase in heart rate and contractility, then blockade of the effect of the sympathetic nervous system is a rational approach to reduce the work load of the heart.

PROPRANOLOL is the prototype agent in this class.

Although propranolol is considered the prototypic β-blocker, there are many other β-blockers that are used. The drugs listed in the table at the beginning of this chapter are FDA-approved for the treatment of angina (propranolol, nadolol, atenolol, and metoprolol).

β-Blockers reduce the frequency and severity of anginal attacks.

β-Blockers are not useful in the treatment of an acute attack of angina. These drugs are generally taken orally on a daily basis to prevent anginal attacks. Use of β-blockers increases the amount of exercise that a patient can tolerate.

ANTIARRHYTHMIC DRUGS

·

Organization of Class

Class I Drugs

Class II Drugs

Class III Drugs

Class IV Drugs

Other Drugs

Final Note

· · · · · · · · · · · ·

ORGANIZATION OF CLASS

Arrhythmias, disturbances of the normal rhythm of the heart, occur when the electrical conduction systems malfunction. The malfunction could result in a change in heart rate, rhythm, impulse generation, or conduction of electrical signals through the heart muscle.

Non-pharmacological approaches to arrhythmias include the use of pacemakers, implantable defibrillators, and ablation of an aberrant conduction pathway.

In order to understand the action and classification of the antiarrhyth-

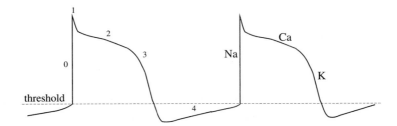

Figure 13-1
The cardiac action potential is shown. The action potential has been divided into phases (indicated on the left). The shape of the action potential is determined by the ions that are flowing during that phase (indicated on the right).

mic drugs, it is necessary to understand the ionic movements that underlie the cardiac action potential (Fig. 13-1).

It is also good to remember the normal flow of electricity in the heart. Who controls the rate? Who controls the rhythm? Who takes over in emergencies?

The antiarrhythmic agents are classified into four groups according to the part of the cardiac cycle that they influence. This is a universal system, but it is not entirely accurate. A number of drugs have more than one effect. There are also agents that do not fall into any of the four categories.

CLASS I DRUGS

> The class I drugs are essentially sodium channel blockers.

The class I drugs are characterized by their ability to block sodium entry into the cell during depolarization. This will decrease the rate of rise of phase 0 of the action potential (Fig. 13-2). These drugs also suppress automaticity of the Purkinje fibers and His bundle. The class I drugs have been further divided into three groups. Class IA drugs slow the rate of rise of phase 0 and prolong the effective refractory period of the ventricle. Class IB drugs have less of an effect on phase 0, but shorten the action potential duration and refractory period of the Purkinje fibers. Class IC drugs have the greatest effect on the early depolarization and have less effect on the refractory period of the ventricle.

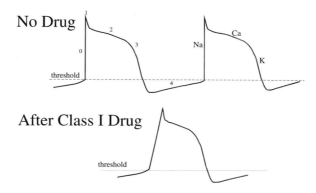

Figure 13-2
Class I antiarrhythmics block sodium entry into myocardial cells during depolarization. This decreases the rate of rise of phase 0.

CLASS IA	**CLASS IB**	**CLASS IC**
QUINIDINE	LIDOCAINE	flecainide
PROCAINAMIDE	phenytoin	propafenone
disopyramide	tocainide	encainide
(moricizine)	mexiletine	indecainide
	(moricizine)	

Here we have a major stumbling block for medical students. Notice that the names of the class I drugs appear to have no rhyme or reason. Depending on whether you have had them yet in class, you may recognize some of the local anesthetics (procainamide and lidocaine). Many of these drugs do sort of look alike, in that they end in *-cainide*. Some serious name recognition drilling will go a long way with this group of drugs.

The names and overall mechanism of action are the most important points for the class I antiarrhythmics. Then you should add a few points about some of the individual agents.

The class IA drugs are useful in the treatment of atrial and ventricular arrhythmias.

These drugs—quinidine, procainamide and disopyramide—are all-purpose antiarrhythmics. Read through the uses and indications for all three and see the similarities. Focus on them. Later go back and consider the differences.

As you might guess from the name, quinidine is related to quinine. Both quinidine and quinine have antimalarial actions (Chap. 34).

The class IB drugs are useful in the treatment of ventricular arrhythmias.

The class IB drugs are much less effective in treating the atrial (supraventricular) arrhythmias as compared with the class IA drugs.

LIDOCAINE is the DRUG OF CHOICE for the treatment of ventricular arrhythmias (ventricular tachycardia, ventricular fibrillation, and ventricular ectopy).

If (or when) you take advanced cardiac life support (ACLS), you will learn how to administer lidocaine in emergency situations. Lidocaine is not as useful in the treatment of atrial arrhythmias.

The class IC agents are useful in suppressing ventricular arrhythmias.

Flecainide and propafenone are absorbed orally and are used for chronic suppression of ventricular arrhythmias (as opposed to acute treatment of ventricular arrhythmias, class IB).

CLASS II DRUGS

The class II antiarrhythmics are β-blockers.

The mechanism of action of these drugs, in terms of rhythm stabilization, is unknown. Use of the β-blockers results in cardiac membrane stabilization. Conduction through the SA and AV nodes is slowed and the refractory period is increased (Fig. 13-3).

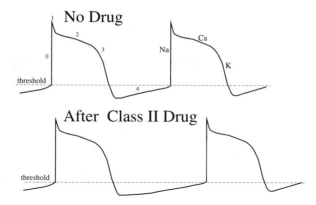

Figure 13-3
Class II antiarrhythmics increase the refractory period between action potentials.

A list of β-blockers is provided in Chap. 12 and in Chap. 10.

These drugs are particularly useful in treating the tachyarrythmias due to increased sympathetic activity.

PROPRANOLOL is the β-blocker most commonly used to treat arrhythmias.

CLASS III DRUGS

The class III antiarrythmics prolong repolarization. They are sometimes designated as potassium channel blockers.

These drugs show complex pharmacological properties. They are classified together because they all prolong the duration of the action potential without altering phase 0 depolarization or the resting membrane potential (Fig. 13-4).

amiodarone
BRETYLIUM
sotalol

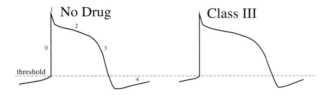

Figure 13-4
Class III antiarrhythmics prolong the duration of the action potential without altering phase 0 depolarization or the resting membrane potential.

It is probably wise to include these drug names in your name recognition list. Be careful not to confuse amiodarone with amrinone (an inotrope). Also, many books do not include sotalol here. You better check your book before you start to memorize anything.

The class III agents are useful in treating intractable ventricular arrhythmias.

CLASS IV DRUGS

The class IV antiarrythmics are the calcium channel blockers.

The calcium channel blockers slow conduction through the AV node and increase the effective refractory period in the AV node.

These actions may terminate reentrant arrhythmias that require the AV node for conduction. A list of calcium channel blockers is provided in Chap. 12. Some of the calcium channel blockers have a greater effect on the heart than the vascular smooth muscle, others are the opposite.

These drugs block the slow, inward calcium current during phases 0 and 2 of the cardiac cycle. By slowing the inward calcium current, these drugs slow conduction and prolong the effective refractory period, especially in the AV node.

> The calcium channel blockers are more effective against atrial than ventricular arrhythmias.

Their side effects are due to other actions of the drugs, such as vasodilation. This should come as no surprise.

OTHER DRUGS

As we said up front, there are a number of drugs that do not neatly fall into the four classes of antiarrythmics.

> Other antiarrhythmic drugs include:
> ADENOSINE
> cardiac glycosides (digoxin)
> magnesium sulfate
> moricizine

> ADENOSINE is the DRUG OF CHOICE for the treatment of parox-ysmal supraventricular tachycardia.

Adenosine is given intravenously and has an exceedingly short half-life (seconds). It depresses AV and sinus node activity. Since the most common form of paroxysmal supraventricular tachycardia involves a reentrant pathway, adenosine is effective in terminating the arrhythmia.

> DIGOXIN is used to control the ventricular rate in atrial fibrillation or flutter.

Digoxin slows conduction through the AV node and increases the refractory period of the AV node. This decreases the number and frequency of impulses that pass from the atria into the ventricle. That's important when the atria is out of control, as in flutterflutter or fibrillation.

> Magnesium sulfate can be effective in terminating refractory ventricular arrhythmias.

Magnesium deficiency is associated with cardiac arrhythmias, cardiac insufficiency, and sudden death. Magnesium replacement can prevent these symptoms of deficiency. This is pretty far down on the trivia list, so if you didn't know it don't worry too much about learning it early on. Save some things to learn later.

> Moricizine prolongs refractory periods.

Moricizine is a relatively new drug that has not found a home (classification-wise) yet. It is sometimes considered a class I agent. Moricizine prolongs the refractory period and decreases conduction in the AV node and Purkinje system.

> Drugs that can be used to increase heart rate include:
> ATROPINE
> ISOPROTERENOL
> EPINEPHRINE

These drugs are used to treat bradycardia. Blocking the parasympathetic system (that tries to slow the heart) with atropine (muscarinic antagonist) will increase the heart rate. For you trivia buffs, a total dose of 3 mg of atropine will produce complete blockade of vagal activity. Sympathetic agonists will also increase heart rate by directly stimulating the β receptors in the heart. The increase in heart rate and contractility can make ischemia worse in a heart at risk.

FINAL NOTE

If you have this material well in hand, you should go back and examine the specific therapy of certain arrhythmias. For example, which drugs are used to treat multifocal atrial tachycardias or Wolff–Parkinson–White? This is when the real fun begins. We will not dive into this morass here, because you have to have the basics before you go into the complexities.

ANTIHYPERTENSIVE DRUGS

·

Organization of Class

Diuretics

Angiotensin-Converting Enzyme (ACE) Inhibitors

Calcium Channel Blockers

Other Vasodilators

α- and β-Blockers

Peripheral Antiadrenergics

Clonidine

· · · · · · · · · · · ·

ORGANIZATION OF CLASS

High blood pressure (hypertension) develops when the blood volume is large compared to the available space in the blood vessels. The control of blood pressure is complex and involves vascular, cardiac, and renal physiology.

Mean arterial pressure = cardiac output × peripheral resistance.

This should be familiar from physiology. From this equation, it is obvious that a decrease in either cardiac output or peripheral resistance will decrease blood pressure. But, the patient has high blood pressure. So, something must have changed one of these factors. A number of factors will increase cardiac output, including increased heart rate, increased contractility, and increased sodium and water retention. Vasoconstriction will increase peripheral resistance. Decreasing one or more of these factors is the goal of antihypertensive therapy. Diuretics can be used to decrease blood volume. Drugs are available that interfere with the renin–angiotensin system, which is intimately involved in salt and water balance in the body. Finally, drugs can be used to decrease peripheral vascular resistance or cardiac output. This can be done with direct-acting vasodilators or by using agents that block sympathetic nervous system output.

I.   Diuretics
   A.   Thiazides
   B.   Loop diuretics
   C.   Potassium-sparing diuretics
II.   Drugs that interfere with the renin–angiotensin system
   A.   ACE inhibitors
   B.   Angiotensin receptor antagonists
III.   Drugs that decrease peripheral vascular resistance or cardiac output
   A.   Direct vasodilators
      1.   Calcium channel blockers
      2.   Others
   B.   Sympathetic nervous system depressants
      1. α-Blockers
      2. β-Blockers
      3.   Centrally active agents
      4.   Others

As you can see, for the antihypertensives it is easiest to organize the drugs by their mechanism of action. Some of these drugs are also useful in the treatment of angina or heart failure. This means that you will see the same drugs more than once. Some students find this confusing. Actually, if you take just a few minutes to compare the drug groups and notice the overlap, it will save you study time in the end. Also, much of cardiovascular pharmacology is a review of autonomic pharmacology.

DIURETICS

Drugs that increase urine flow are called *diuretics*. Diuretics play an important role in the management of high blood pressure. They are often used in combination with other classes of antihypertensive drugs. These drugs are ion transport inhibitors in the kidney, so a short review of renal physiology may be useful for you at this point.

There are basically three groups of diuretics, named by structure and mechanism of action. Consider the group names for a second. Notice the potassium-sparing group. This should tell you that the other two groups cause a loss of potassium. You now know a major side effect of both the thiazide diuretics and the loop diuretics. Next consider the name "loop diuretics." If you had to guess the site of action of these drugs, what would you guess? I hope you said the loop of Henle. So you already know the site of action of that group (Fig. 14-1).

THIAZIDE DIURETICS	LOOP DIURETICS	K$^+$-SPARING DIURETICS
CHLOROTHIAZIDE HYDROCHLORO-THIAZIDE	FUROSEMIDE bumetanide	SPIRONOLACTONE amiloride
metolazone chlorthalidone	ethacrynic acid muzolimine	triamterene indapamide

Name recognition is extremely important here. Many a student has missed an exam (or board) question because they didn't recognize drug X

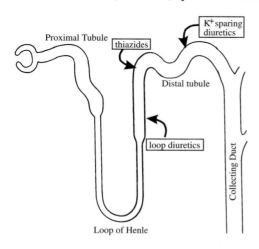

Figure 14-1
The location of action of the different classes of diuretics is illustrated here. The loop diuretics act in the ascending loop of Henle. The thiazide diuretics and potassium-(K$^+$) sparing diuretics act in the distal tubule.

as a K$^+$-sparing diuretic. This is made more difficult by the fact that the names do not have similar endings (or beginnings).

The thiazide diuretics inhibit sodium and chloride reabsorption in the thick ascending loop of Henle and early distal tubule. This loss of ions increases urine volume.

The thiazide diuretics are the DRUGS OF CHOICE in the treatment of primary hypertension.

Primary hypertension is high blood pressure for which no cause can be found. High blood pressure can be secondary to many things, including renal artery stenosis, tumors of the adrenal gland, and so on. Primary hypertension is not secondary to any identifiable cause. The thiazide diuretics are not recommended in patients with renal insufficiency.

The thiazide diuretics can cause hypokalemia.

But, you already know this, don't you?! Remember, there are potassium-sparing diuretics and they aren't thiazides.

The loop diuretics inhibit chloride reabsorption in the thick ascending loop of Henle.

The action in the loop of Henle gives them their name "loop diuretics." So, you only need to add the chloride reabsorption part.

The loop diuretics are the DRUGS OF CHOICE for reducing pulmonary edema in congestive heart failure.

The use of the loop diuretics in the treatment of pulmonary edema is because of their high potency and rapid onset of action.

The major side effect of the loop diuretics is hypokalemia.

Nothing new here!! The loop diuretics are more potent than the thiazide diuretics. They are the preferred diuretics in patients with low glomerular filtration rates. They can cause a host of metabolic abnormalities, the most common being hypokalemia (low K^+). Dehydration can also be a problem. They can increase the toxicity of drugs that cause ototoxicity (ear) and nephrotoxicity (kidney).

The K^+-sparing diuretics enhance sodium excretion and retain potassium by an action in the distal tubule.

SPIRONOLACTONE is an antagonist of aldosterone (which causes sodium retention).

The potassium-sparing diuretics are often used in combination with the other diuretics to help with the potassium balance. They can cause hyperkalemia. Alone, the K^+-sparing diuretics are not very potent.

ANGIOTENSIN-CONVERTING ENZYME (ACE) INHIBITORS

These drugs were discussed in Chap. 11 because they are useful in the treatment of heart failure. Their action in the treatment of hypertension is also due to their vasodilating effects. Most of this information is, therefore, duplicative from Chap. 11. That's what makes this stuff easier.

CAPTOPRIL	benazepril
lisinopril	fosinopril
pentapril	quinapril
ramipril	ENALAPRIL

As always, check the names in the table against the ones in your textbook or class handouts and make any corrections necessary. These drugs are relatively recent developments and new ones are appearing on a regular basis. Hopefully the *-pril* ending will continue to be used; it makes these drugs very easy to identify.

Angiotensin I is converted to angiotensin II by the enzyme angiotensin-converting enzyme (ACE), which is also called peptidyl-dipeptidase. Angiotensin II is a potent vasoconstrictor and stimulator of aldosterone secretion. Aldosterone promotes sodium and water retention and potassium excretion. This leads to an increase in vascular volume and an increase in peripheral vascular resistance.

> The ACE inhibitors block the conversion of angiotensin I to angiotensin II.

With less angiotensin II around there is less vasoconstriction and less aldosterone production. This leads to a decrease in peripheral vascular resistance. This should be old hat by now. (I could have left this out, but sometimes it's nice to see something that you already know).

> The major side effects of the ACE inhibitors are related to the hypotensive action of the drugs—headache, dizziness, tachycardia, and so on.

As we saw with the nitrates and calcium channel blockers, drugs that cause vasodilatation cause side effects directly related to the vasodilatation. The tachycardia is a reflex increase in heart rate in response to the decrease in blood pressure. These drugs are particularly useful in hypertension that is due to increased renin levels. The ACE inhibitors do not affect glucose levels, so they are also used in patients with diabetes.

> Saralasin is an angiotensin receptor blocking agent.

Saralasin is not an ACE inhibitor, but is mentioned here because if you associate it with the ACE inhibitors you are more likely to remember what it is. Saralasin must be given intravenously. A new orally active angiotensin II receptor antagonist, losartan, just appeared on the market.

CALCIUM CHANNEL BLOCKERS

> Calcium channel blockers are used to treat hypertension because they produce vasodilation.

I hope that you knew that one!!! The calcium channel blockers were introduced in Chap. 12 as antianginal agents. They block the entry of calcium into cells. When the cell is a muscle cell of a blood vessel wall, then the cell can no longer contract. This blockade of contraction leads to vasodilation. Individual agents are listed in Chap. 12.

OTHER VASODILATORS

There are several other agents that act directly on smooth muscle cells and result in vasodilation. For these other drugs, name recognition as vasodilators is the most important thing for you to focus on.

> Hydralazine, minoxidil, and pinacidil directly relax arterioles.

The arteriole relaxation results in a decrease in blood pressure, but the exact mechanism of action of these drugs is not clear. The decrease in blood pressure leads to reflex tachycardia and increased cardiac output (not good in a patient with limited cardiac reserve). These drugs will also increase plasma renin concentration. The reflex tachycardia can be blocked with β-blockers. Diuretics can be used to counter the sodium and water retention.

An aside: Minoxidil causes unwanted hair growth in patients receiving the drug for the treatment of hypertension. The drug is also marketed for topical treatment of baldness. I presume that you have seen the TV commercials for minoxidil (ROGAINE).

> Diazoxide is a vasodilator used for hypertensive emergencies.

Diazoxide is used in the hospital setting to produce a decrease in blood pressure during hypertensive emergencies. It also suppresses insulin release and increases hepatic glucose release. This results in an increase in plasma glucose levels.

NITROPRUSSIDE is a vasodilator given by continuous intravenous infusion. It is rapidly metabolized to cyanide.

The mechanism of nitroprusside is similar to that of the nitrates (Chap. 12). Nitroprusside is used in hypertensive emergencies to rapidly bring down a dangerously high blood pressure. The blood pressure can be controlled with small changes in the IV infusion rate.

α- AND β-BLOCKERS

The α_1 antagonists, such as PRAZOSIN, terazosin, and doxazosin, will dilate arteries and veins.

Remember from autonomics that blood vessels are primarily under α-receptor control. α Agonists cause vasoconstriction and α antagonists cause vasodilation. Therefore, the use of α antagonists makes sense for the treatment of hypertension. The mixed α_1, β_1, and β_2 antagonist, labetalol, dilates blood vessels (α_1) without causing an reflex increase in heart rate (β_1).

β-Blockers prevent sympathetic stimulation of the heart.

β-blockers have some use in the treatment of hypertension. They decrease heart rate and cardiac output (β_1) and will decrease renin release (β_1).

Some β-blockers that can be used to treat hypertension include:
  atenolol (β_1)
  betaxolol (β_1)
  carteolol (β_1)
  penbutolol (β_1)
  metaprolol (β_1)
  acebutolol (β_1 plus some sympathomimetic activity)
  esmolol (β_1 plus some sympathomimetic activity)
  PROPRANOLOL (β_1 and β_2)
  nadolol (β_1 and β_2)
  timolol (β_1 and β_2)
  pindolol (β_1 and β_2 plus some sympathomimetic activity)

As you can see from the list, both β_1 selective and nonselective blockers have been successfully used in the treatment of hypertension.

PERIPHERAL ANTI-ADRENERGICS

There are other drugs that influence the action of the sympathetic nervous system. These are less important in the treatment of hypertension than the α- and β-blockers, so you can defer the names and mechanisms here if you are really strapped for time and energy right now.

Reserpine depletes catecholamine stores.

The depletion of catecholamine stores by reserpine results in a decrease in total peripheral resistance, heart rate, and cardiac output. The action of reserpine leaves the parasympathetic nervous system in charge.

Guanethidine and guanadrel deplete norepinephrine from terminals and interferes with release.

These drugs are antihypertensive because they prevent the release of neurotransmitter from the postganglionic sympathetic nerves.

CLONIDINE

Reduction of sympathetic outflow will result in a net decrease in blood pressure. Three drugs are active centrally: clonidine, methyldopa (or α-methyldopa), and guanabenz. Go for name recognition as centrally active agents that reduce sympathetic outflow.

CLONIDINE and guanabenz are α_2 agonists that reduce central sympathetic outflow. Methyldopa also reduces sympathetic outflow by a central action.

These drugs will decrease total peripheral resistance without changing cardiac output. As you would predict, these drugs have no direct effect on the kidney and can be used in patients with renal disease. The side effects of these drugs include drowsiness and dry mouth (sounds like anticholinergic actions to me). There are some differences in the mechanism of action of these compounds.

An aside: Be careful not to confuse guanabenz with guanethidine or guanadrel. They can all be used to treat hypertension, but have different mechanisms.

DRUGS THAT AFFECT THE BLOOD

·

Organization of Class

Anticoagulants

Antiplatelet Agents

Thrombolytic or Fibrinolytic Drugs

Antianemia Drugs

· · · · · · · · · · · ·

ORGANIZATION OF CLASS

The processes of hemostasis consist of three phases: vascular, platelet, and coagulation (Fig. 15-1). The fibrinolytic phase prevents the clotting process from spreading out of control beyond the site of injury. This would be a great time for you to review hemostatic mechanisms in your physiology textbook.

Platelets respond to tissue injury by adhesion to the site of injury; they then release granules containing chemical mediators that promote aggregation. Factors released by platelets and the injured tissue cause activation of

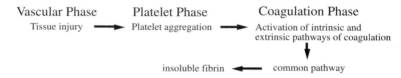

Figure 15-1
Hemostasis consists of three phases: vascular, platelet, and coagulation. The end result of the three phases is the formation of fibrin.

the coagulation cascade. This results in the formation of thrombin, which in turn converts fibrinogen to fibrin. The subsequent cross-linking of the fibrin strands stabilizes the clot.

Drugs are available that will interfere with the platelet and coagulation phases of the initial response to tissue injury.

Anticoagulant drugs
  HEPARIN
  WARFARIN
  dicumarol
  anisindion
Antiplatelet drugs
  ASPIRIN
  DIPYRIDAMOLE
  sulfinpyrazone
  ticlopidine
  abciximab
Thrombolytic drugs/fibrinogen activators
  STREPTOKINASE
  urokinase
  t-PA
  anistreplase

Compare the drugs in this table to those in your textbook or class handouts. Cross off any that you do not need to learn and add any new ones. Watch for name changes too.

As we go through the drugs that prevent clots and the drugs that lyse clots, the drugs that can function as antidotes will be mentioned. Finally we will consider drugs used to treat anemia.

Treatment of bleeding (antidote for . . .)
   aminocaproic acid (thrombolytic)
   tranexamic acid (thrombolytic)
   PROTAMINE SULFATE (heparin)
   Vitamin K (oral anticoagulants)
Treatment of anemia
  IRON
  folic acid;
  cyanocobalamin (B_{12})
  ERYTHROPOIETIN
  epoetin alpha

The drugs listed for the treatment of bleeding are essentially antidotes for the drugs used to prevent clotting or to lyse clots. For example, protamine sulfate is an antidote for heparin.

ANTICOAGULANTS

Anticoagulant drugs inhibit the development and enlargement of clots. It should be obvious from the name of the group that the drugs act by interfering with the coagulation phase of hemostasis. These drugs are normally divided into heparin and the others. The others are orally active and include warfarin and dicumarol.

The major side effect of all of the anticoagulants is hemorrhage.

This should be intuitive, but it warrants a mention.

Anticoagulant drugs are NOT effective against clots that have already formed.

Anticoagulant therapy provides prophylaxis against venous and arterial thrombosis. They cannot dissolve clots that have already formed, but may prevent or slow extension of an existing clot. They are useful in preventing deep vein thrombosis and pulmonary embolism. Anticoagulation of patients with atrial fibrillation has reduced the risk of systemic embolism and stroke.

> HEPARIN binds to antithrombin III and accelerates the interaction of antithrombin III to the coagulation factors.

The binding of antithrombin III to the coagulation factors prevents them from taking part in coagulation (Fig. 15-2). This is easy to remember from the names. Antithrombin is against (anti) thrombin, which is trying to thrombose (clot).

> HEPARIN must be given parenterally (intravenously or subcutaneously).

By referring to the anticoagulants as heparin and the oral agents, it should be obvious that heparin cannot be given orally. In fact, heparin does not cross membranes very well at all. If given intravenously, it has an almost immediate anticoagulant effect.

> PROTAMINE is a specific heparin antagonist that can be used to treat heparin-induced hemorrhage.

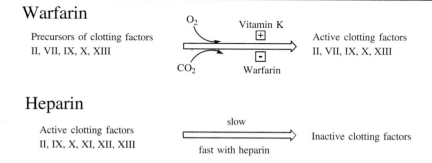

Figure 15-2
Just as a visual reminder, this figure shows warfarin blocking the activation of clotting factors, and heparin speeding the inactivation of clotting factors.

Protamines are basic proteins that have a high affinity for the negatively charged heparin. The binding of protamine and heparin is immediate and results in an inert complex.

The oral anticoagulants are vitamin K antagonists.

Before they can participate in the clotting process, several of the protein coagulation factors require vitamin K for their activation. The oral anticoagulants interfere with this action of vitamin K. Therefore, the oral anticoagulants delay activation of new coagulation factors (Fig. 15.2). They do not affect the factors that have already been activated. These means there is a delay in the onset of action of the oral anticoagulants. So, if a patient comes in with an acute clot in the leg that is threatening to break loose, do you initiate therapy with warfarin or heparin? I hope you said heparin—for its immediate action.

Administration of vitamin K can overcome the anticoagulant effects of the oral agents, but the effect takes about 24 hours.

The time it takes for vitamin K to overcome the anticoagulant effects of the oral agents is also directly related to the mechanism of action. It takes time to make new coagulation factors.

WARFARIN is the oral anticoagulant of choice.

The oral anticoagulants are used when long-term therapy is indicated.

There are a large number of drug interactions with the oral anticoagulants.

There are many drugs that both increase and decrease the effect of the oral anticoagulants. It is not possible to memorize them all. The important thing for now is to remember that there are lots of drug interactions.

ANTIPLATELET AGENTS

Platelet aggregation inhibitors decrease the formation of chemical signals that promote platelet aggregation. Drugs that inhibit platelet function are administered for the relatively specific *prophylaxis* of arterial thrombosis and during management of heart attacks (myocardial infarction).

ASPIRIN inhibits platelet aggregation and will prolong bleeding time.

Aspirin will be considered in more detail later (Chap. 43). It irreversibly inhibits cyclooxygenase. In platelets this inhibits the formation of TxA_2 (a thromboxane). Recall that platelets do not have a nucleus and cannot make more of the enzyme after aspirin irreversible inhibits it. The cyclooxygenase in endothelial cells is also inhibited, but they can make more enzyme.

DIPYRIDAMOLE decreases platelet adhesion to damaged endothelium, but does not alter bleeding time.

Dipyridamole is a phosphodiesterase inhibitor and increases cAMP levels in platelets. It is reported also to be a coronary vasodilator (antianginal). It is usually used in combination with aspirin or warfarin.

Sulfinpyrazone and ticlopidine are two other agents that can act as antiplatelet drugs. Sulfinpyrazone is an NSAID that competitively inhibits cyclooxygenase, and it is used to treat gout because it blocks reuptake of uric acid in the kidney. It also happens to inhibit platelet function. Ticlopidine inhibits platelet aggregation and prolongs bleeding time, but its mechanism of action is not understood.

An aside: Be careful with some of the drugs that start with sulf. They are easily confused. For example, I often confuse sulfinpyrazone with sulfasalazine (used to treat Crohn's disease, Chap. 42).

Recently, a monoclonal antibody to platelet glycoprotein became available. It prevents platelet aggregation. The drug name is abciximab.

THROMBOLYTIC OR FIBRINOLYTIC DRUGS

> Anticoagulant and antiplatelet drugs are administered to prevent the formation of clots. Thrombolytic drugs are used to lyse already formed clots.

This is an important distinction for the clinical use of these various drugs.

Fibrinolysis is the process of breaking down the fibrin that holds the clot together. Fibrinolysis is initiated by the activation of plasminogen to plasmin. The plasmin then catalyzes the degradation of fibrin. The activation of plasminogen is normally initiated by plasminogen activators (aren't these names hard? for once they are named for their job!).

> The thrombolytic drugs are plasminogen activators.

There are currently two generations of plasminogen activators: first and second. The first generation drugs (streptokinase and urokinase) convert all plasminogen to plasmin throughout the plasma. The second generation drugs (t-PA) selectively activate plasminogen bound to fibrin. This is supposed to reduce the side effects of the drug by targeting the site of action.

> Clot dissolution and reperfusion is more likely if therapy is initiated early after clot formation. Clots become more difficult to lyse as they age.

Thrombolytic drugs have been shown to lyse clots in arteries and veins and to reestablish tissue perfusion. They are used in the management of pulmonary embolism, deep vein thrombosis, and arterial thromboembolism. They have proven to be particularly useful in acute heart attack due to a clot in a coronary artery.

> The main side effect of the thrombolytic drugs is bleeding.

This should not come as a surprise to you.

> STREPTOKINASE is a foreign protein and is antigenic. t-PA is not antigenic.

Because of its antigenicity, one of the side effects of streptokinase is an allergic-anaphylactic reaction. Patients may also develop antibodies to streptokinase and inactivate it. These reactions are less likely to occur after t-PA administration.

> Anistreplase is also known as acetylated streptokinase–plasminogen activator complex (ASPAC) and it consists of a complex of strepto-kinase and plasminogen.

Because it contains streptokinase, anistreplase has the same problems as streptokinase. However, it has a longer duration of action as compared with streptokinase.

> Aminocaproic acid and tranexamic acid are antifibrinolytic drugs and can function as antidotes for the thrombolytic drugs.

ANTIANEMIA DRUGS

Anemia is defined as a plasma hemoglobin level that is below normal. It can be due to a decreased number of circulating red blood cells or an abnormally low total hemoglobin content. There are many causes of anemia. Before treatment, the cause needs to be determined.

> Iron salts, such as ferrous sulfate, are used as iron supplements to treat iron deficiency anemia.

Folic acid deficiency leads to megaloblastic anemia.

Deficiency of vitamin B_{12} also indirectly leads to megaloblastic anemia. Administration of folate without B_{12} will correct the anemia, but will not correct the neurologic dysfunction due to lack of B_{12}.

Pernicious anemia is due to a loss of intrinsic factor, which results in a deficiency of vitamin B_{12}.

ERYTHROPOIETIN is synthesized in the kidney in response to hypoxia or anemia. It then stimulates erythropoiesis (red cell proliferation).

Epoetin alpha is human recombinant erythropoietin.

Human erythropoietin is used in the treatment of anemia associated with end-stage renal failure.

LIPID-LOWERING DRUGS

·

Organization of Class

Some Additional Explanation of Mechanisms

· · · · · · · · · · · ·

ORGANIZATION OF CLASS

Coronary heart disease, heart attacks, and strokes have been shown to be correlated with plasma levels of serum cholesterol and lipoprotein particles. Therefore, there has been increased interest in lowering the cholesterol and lipoprotein levels in patients by diet or by pharmacological intervention.

Drugs used in the treatment of elevated serum lipids (hyperlipidemias) are targeted to decrease production of lipoprotein or cholesterol, increase degradation of a lipoprotein, or increase removal of cholesterol from the body. The lipoproteins are proteins that bind and transport fats, such as lipids and triglycerides, around in the blood. They are classified according to lipid and protein content, transport function, and mechanism of lipid delivery. The high density lipoproteins (HDL) are considered the "good guys" as compared with the low- and very-low-density lipoproteins (LDL and VLDL).

The most important facts about the relatively few drugs in this class are the mechanisms of action. Practically speaking, taste, bulk needed to be consumed, and cost are important considerations.

DRUGS	MECHANISM
colestipol CHOLESTYRAMINE	Bile acid binding resins
niacin	?
LOVASTATIN pravastatin fluvastatin simvastatin	Inhibit HMG CoA reductase
gemfibrozil	Inhibits VLDL synthesis Increases lipoprotein lipase activity
clofibrate	Increases lipoprotein lipase activity
probucol	Increases LDL degradation and cholesterol excretion

First of all, compare the list of drugs in the table with the ones in your textbook or class handouts. Add or delete drugs as needed. Then compare the mechanisms of action to those that you have. Some of these are not entirely worked out so there may be discrepancies. Do not let that throw you off.

Basically, the table above is the most important stuff to know. If it is too much for you to start with, learn the two bile-binding resins and the -*statins* (or -*vastatins*) that inhibit HMG CoA reductase. The rest of the drugs alter metabolism of lipoproteins. If you are doing great, skip the rest of this chapter.

SOME ADDITIONAL EXPLANATION OF MECHANISMS

The bile-binding resins (cholestyramine and colestipol) are anion exchange resins that bind negatively charged bile acids in the small intestine. The resins are not absorbed and are not metabolized. The resin–bile acid complex is excreted in the feces (Fig. 16-1). The body compensates for the reduction in bile acids by converting cholesterol to bile acids, thus effectively lowering the cholesterol levels. Because of the mechanism of action, it should seem reasonable to you that these resins may also affect the absorption of other drugs and the fat soluble vitamins.

The -*statins* contain structural analogues of 3-hydroxy-3-methyl-glutarate (HMG), which is a precursor of cholesterol. They inhibit HMG

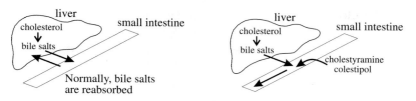

Figure 16-1
Normally, bile acids are secreted into the small intestine and then reabsorbed almost completely. Cholestyramine and colestipol bind to the bile acids in the small intestine and prevent their reabsoprtion. This causes the liver to use cholesterol to make more bile acids.

CoA reductase, the enzyme that controls the rate-limiting step in cholesterol synthesis. This will deplete intracellular cholesterol. The cell then looks to the extracellular space for the cholesterol it needs. This results in a lowering of the plasma cholesterol levels.

Niacin lowers both plasma cholesterol and triglyceride levels. The lipid-lowering effects are due to decreased hepatic secretion of VLDL. This appears to be due to decreased triglyceride synthesis.

Probucil alters the structure of LDL. The "new" LDL is removed from the plasma faster than normal LDL.

DRUGS ACTING ON THE CENTRAL NERVOUS SYSTEM

·

DRUGS USED IN PARKINSON'S DISEASE

·

Class Organization

Dopamine Replacement Therapy

Dopamine Agonist Therapy

Anticholinergic Therapy

· · · · · · · · · · · ·

CLASS ORGANIZATION

In this case the drugs are arranged by mechanism of action. The groups are quite easy to remember if you remember the pathology of Parkinson's Disease.

In Parkinson's disease there is a loss of the dopamine-containing neurons in the substantia nigra (Fig. 17-1). These neurons normally project to the caudate putamen (one piece of the basal ganglia) where the dopamine inhibits firing of the cholinergic neurons. These cholinergic neurons form excitatory synapses onto other neurons that project out of the basal ganglia. The result of the loss of dopamine neurons is that the cholinergic neurons are now without their normal inhibition—sort of like a car going down a hill without any brakes.

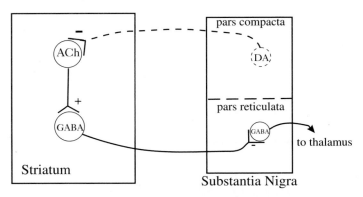

Figure 17-1
Diagram of projections into and out of the striatum. In Parkinson's disease there is a loss of the dopamine-(DA) containing neurons that project from the substantia nigra to the striatum, where they inhibit cholinergic (ACh) neurons (dashed line).

Therapy for Parkinson's:
1. Dopamine replacement therapy
2. Dopamine agonist therapy
3. Anticholinergic therapy

The goals of therapy are to correct the imbalance of the cholinergic neurons in the striatum. All of the therapeutic approaches to Parkinson's disease "make sense." Given the loss of dopamine containing neurons, you could replace the dopamine or give dopamine agonists (to mimic the action of the lost dopamine). Given the "uninhibited" cholinergic neurons you could give an anticholinergic to try and restore inhibition. If you can remember this much you are well on your way to a good grasp of this area.

DOPAMINE REPLACEMENT THERAPY

It would be nice if we could just give dopamine itself. However, dopamine will not cross the blood–brain barrier (Fig. 17-2).

LEVODOPA (L-DOPA) is a metabolic precursor of dopamine that crosses the blood–brain barrier.

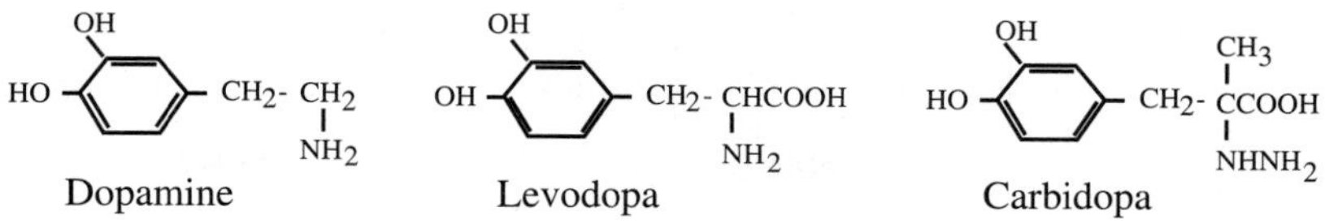

Figure 17-2
Structures of dopamine, levodopa, and carbidopa

Large doses of levodopa are required because much of the drug is decarboxylated to dopamine in the periphery. All this dopamine floating around peripherally causes side effects.

CARBIDOPA is a dopamine decarboxylase inhibitor that does not cross the blood–brain barrier. It reduces the peripheral metabolism of levodopa, thereby increasing the amount of levodopa that reaches the brain.

Carbidopa and levodopa are used today in combination. This is a prime example of a GOOD drug interaction that is logical based on the mechanisms.

Side effects of levodopa and carbidopa are related to the dopamine that is generated by peripheral decarboxylation (the carbidopa is not perfect).

DOPAMINE AGONIST THERAPY

The theory behind the use of dopamine agonists is that the dopamine-releasing neurons have disappeared, but the postsynaptic dopamine receptors are still present and functional. Administration of dopamine agonists to stimulate these receptors would then restore the balance of inhibition and excitation in the basal ganglia.

The main role of these drugs is in combination with levodopa and carbidopa in early Parkinson's disease.

Bromocriptine and pergolide are two dopamine agonists used in the treatment of Parkinson's disease.

The actions and side effects of these drugs are similar to levodopa. Warning: For those of you who are heroic and have decided to memorize the structures of these drugs, both of these drugs are ergotamine derivatives and are quite complex.

SELEGILINE, a.k.a DEPRENYL, is an inhibitor of MAO-B, the enzyme that metabolizes dopamine in the CNS.

Selegiline is also known as deprenyl. They cannot seem to decide on the correct name for this compound and both names appear in books and articles in the medical literature. This is not a ploy to increase the difficulty of pharmacology for students. Inhibiting MAO-B slows the breakdown of dopamine, thus dopamine remains in the vicinity of its receptors on the cholinergic neurons for a longer period of time. Obviously, you should use caution when using this drug together with levodopa.

ANTICHOLINERGIC THERAPY

Anticholinergic agents are less commonly used, but always taught in pharmacology courses. They reduce the effectiveness of the "uninhibited" cholinergic neurons in the basal ganglia. These drugs are muscarinic antagonists and only differ in potency. Having learned autonomic pharmacology, you should be able to list the side effects of muscarinic antagonists. Therefore, there is really little new here. However, the drug names are quite awkward and easily unrecognizable as antimuscarinic agents.

Trihexylphenidyl, benztropine, and biperiden are muscarinic antagonists used in Parkinson's disease.

Side effects of the above drugs include dry mouth, constipation, urinary retention, and confusion.

Bromocriptine, pergolide, trihexylphenidyl, benztropine, and biperiden are good candidates for your drug name recognition list.

ANXIOLYTIC AND HYPNOTIC DRUGS

·

Tolerance and Dependence

Class Organization

Barbiturates

Benzodiazepines

Other Drugs

· · · · · · · · · · · · ·

TOLERANCE AND DEPENDENCE

At some point before we get into the CNS sedatives and narcotics, we need to make sure about a few terms and definitions.

> *Tolerance* is characterized by a reduced drug effect with repeated use of the drug. Higher doses are needed to produce the same effect.

Essentially, tolerance is reduced effectiveness. The term does not give any indication of the mechanism. Tolerance could be due to increased elimination of the drug or to reduced effectiveness of the drug–receptor interaction. For some drugs, tolerance will develop to one effect of the drug and not to other effects. For example, with the narcotics, tolerance to the analgesic effect is seen, but less tolerance develops to the respiratory depression.

Cross-tolerance means that individuals tolerant to one drug will be tolerant to other drugs in the same class, but not to drugs in other classes.

A person who is tolerant to the sedative effects of one barbiturate will be tolerant to the effect of all the barbiturates (cross-tolerance). However, that person will not be tolerant to the sedative effects of opiates.

Dependence is characterized by withdrawal signs and symptoms.

Dependence can be physical, in which case the person has physical signs of withdrawal, or it can be psychological, in which case the person has psychological signs of withdrawal. There is a thing called cross-dependence, which is similar to cross-tolerance.

CLASS ORGANIZATION

Drugs that are classified as anxiolytics and hypnotics are used for a variety of purposes, including treatment of anxiety and epilepsy, sleep induction, and anesthesia. They are often called sedative-hypnotics or just anxiolytics.

Cross-tolerance and cross-dependence occur between all of the CNS sedatives, including the barbiturates, benzodiazepines, and ethanol.

This is an important feature of all the drugs in this class.

These drugs are generally classified by chemical structure. The two largest groups of drugs are the barbiturates and benzodiazepines. There are a relatively large number of drugs in both of these groups, but (thankfully) their names are generally recognizable.

BARBITURATES	BENZODIAZEPINES	OTHERS
PHENOBARBITAL	DIAZEPAM	buspirone
PENTOBARBITAL	CHLORDIAZEPOXIDE	chloralhydrate
secobarbital	flurazepam	meprobamate
amobarbital	ALPRAZOLAM	
THIOPENTAL	LORAZEPAM	
methohexital	temazepam	
	triazolam	
	quazepam	
	clonazepam	
	clorazepate	
	oxazepam	

Notice that the barbiturates all end in *-tal,* and all, EXCEPT for thiopental and methohexital, end in *-barbital.* The benzodiazepines end in *-pam* or *-lam* for the most part. The notable exception here is chlordiazepoxide. This makes it easy to succeed at name recognition.

All of these drugs will reduce anxiety at low doses and produce sedation at slightly higher doses (Fig. 18-1). Most will induce sleep (hypnosis), thus the name sedative-hypnotics. At higher doses the barbiturates will produce some degree of anesthesia and at even higher doses will produce medullary depression and death.

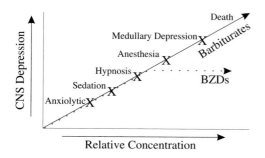

Figure 18-1
This graph schematizes the effects of the benzodiazepines (BZDs) and barbiturates. Notice that the effect of the barbiturates continue up the line of CNS depression to death, while the benzodiazepines veer off after hypnosis.

BARBITURATES

Barbiturates enhance the function of GABA in the CNS.

Barbiturates both enhance GABA responses and mimic GABA by opening the Cl⁻ channel in the absence of GABA. Some barbiturates enhance GABA more than they mimic GABA and others lean more the other way. The net result of both actions is an increase in inhibition in the CNS.

Barbiturates will:
1. Produce sedation, hypnosis, coma, and DEATH
2. Suppress respiration (overdose can lead to DEATH)
3. Induce the liver P-450 system

All the barbiturates will suppress respiration by inhibiting the hypoxic and CO_2 response of the chemoreceptors. This means that a slight increase in the CO_2 content of the blood does not result in an increase in respiration when the patient has taken barbiturates.

Any other drug that is metabolized by the P-450 system will be altered by the presence of barbiturates.

All the barbiturates are liver-metabolized and *all* will induce the cytochrome P-450 microsomal enzymes. Thus, there are a whole list of drug interactions for the barbiturates.

The selection of a particular barbiturate depends on the duration of action of the agent, which depends on the lipid solubility.

The barbiturates are classified according to their duration of action. Thiopental is ultra-short acting (minutes), pentobarbital, secobarbital, and amobarbital are short-acting (hours), and phenobarbital is long-acting (days). Thiopental (ultra-short acting) is highly lipid soluble. After administration it rapidly enters the brain and then is redistributed into other body tissues and eventually into fat. As it redistributes, the concentration in the brain drops below effective levels. Therefore, the duration of action of thiopental is very short.

At this point some students try to memorize the duration of action of the barbiturates. Basically either memorize the duration of action or the use, but not both (since they are connected). All the ultra-short-acting barbiturates are used in anesthesia (see Chap. 23). The long duration barbiturate (phenobarbital) is used to treat epilepsy (see Chap. 21).

> Symptoms of withdrawal in a person dependent on barbiturates include anxiety, nausea and vomiting, hypotension, seizures, and psychosis. Cardiovascular collapse may develop, leading to DEATH.

Physical dependence on barbiturates develops with chronic use. The symptoms of barbiturate withdrawal can be quite serious and even FATAL.

BENZODIAZEPINES

Benzodiazepines are the most widely used anxiolytic drugs because they are relatively safe and effective.

> Benzodiazepines bind to a specific site associated with the $GABA_A$ receptor, which results in increased inhibition.

Binding of benzodiazepines to this specific site enhances the affinity of GABA receptors for GABA, resulting in more frequent opening of the chloride channels. The increased influx of chloride causes hyperpolarization and increased inhibition.

All benzodiazepines reduce anxiety and produce sedation. In contrast to the barbiturates, the benzodiazepines reduce anxiety at doses that do not produce sedation. Some agents are used as antiepileptic agents and some are used in the induction of anesthesia. Duration of action and pharmacokinetic properties are important in selecting the drug to use.

> Most benzodiazepines are metabolized in the liver to active metabolites. In general, the metabolites have slower elimination rates than the parent compound.

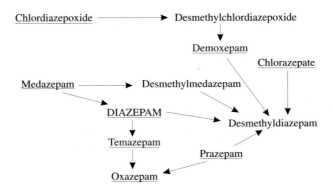

Figure 18-2
The metabolism and interrelationship of many of the benzodiazepines are shown in this figure. The compounds that are available pharmacological preparations are underlined.

It is not necessary to memorize a metabolism scheme for benzodiazepines. However, glance at Fig. 18-2 and notice that many of the agents in this class appear to be interrelated.

There are a few benzodiazepines that are NOT extensively metabolized. They tend to have shorter half-lives.

This issue of elimination half-life for the benzodiazepines can be confusing. Some books are not real clear about whether they indicate the half-life of the parent compound only or the total half-life of the parent plus the active metabolites.

Elimination half-life is not the same as duration of action for the benzodiazepines.

The elimination half-life is determined by the rate of liver metabolism and/or renal excretion. In other words, the half-life measures the time that the drug is present in the body. It says nothing about the time that the drug is present at the GABA receptors in the brain, which gives the duration of action. A drug may spend days hiding from the liver microsomal enzymes in a fat pad. This drug would have a very long elimination half-life and a short duration of action, since while it's in hiding it has no action on the brain (Fig. 18-3).

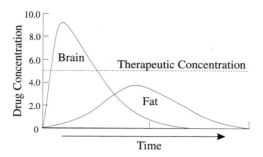

Figure 18-3
This graph shows the change in brain and fat levels of a benzodiazepine after a single administration. The brain levels rise quickly because of the high lipid-solubility of the drug and the high perfusion rate of the brain. The levels in fat increase more slowly because of the much lower perfusion rate of fat. None of the drug in this graph has undergone liver metabolism or renal excretion. Therefore, the duration of action is much shorter than the elimination of half-life.

Physical and psychological dependence to benzodiazepines can occur.

Withdrawal from benzodiazepines can appear as confusion, anxiety, agitation, and restlessness. Benzodiazepines with short half-lives induce more abrupt and severe withdrawal reactions than drugs with longer half-lives.

FLUMAZENIL is a benzodiazepine antagonist.

Flumazenil can be used to reverse the sedative effects of benzo-diazepines after anesthesia or after overdose with benzodiazepines.

It may be useful to add some specific facts about the use of individual agents to the general knowledge we have reviewed so far.

Some specific benzodiazepines have special uses.
DIAZEPAM: muscle relaxation and treatment of status epilepticus
CHLORDIAZEPOXIDE: alcohol withdrawal

> Temazepam, triazolam, and flurazepam are marketed for sleep.

You can remember the first two because they are the two that start with T.

> ALPRAZOLAM is the most commonly prescribed benzodiazepine for anxiety.

Over the years different benzodiazepines have been preferred for the treatment of anxiety. The current reigning favorite is alprazolam. You can use the A to help you remember anxiety.

OTHER DRUGS

> BUSPIRONE is a non-benzodiazepine that is used as an anxiolytic.

Buspirone is relatively nonsedating and has few CNS side effects. It's mechanism of action is unknown, but it may act as a serotonin receptor agonist. Zolpidem is a new agent that you may also hear about.

> Zolpidem is a new non-benzodiazepine agent that is marketed for sleep.

ANTIDEPRESSANTS AND LITHIUM (DRUGS USED TO TREAT MOOD DISORDERS)

·

Class Organization

Heterocyclics

Serotonin-Specific Reuptake Inhibitors (SSRIs)

Monoamine Oxidase (MAO) Inhibitors

Lithium

·　·　·　·　·　·　·　·　·　·　·　·

CLASS ORGANIZATION

It is best to divide the antidepressants into three groups. One, the heterocyclics, consists mostly of tricyclic compounds. They are grouped together mostly based on structure, but they all have similar actions and side effects. The other two groups are based on their mechanism of action. Therefore, if you can remember the name of the group, you have already learned an important fact about each drug in the group.

The trouble most students seem to have with these drugs is their names. Look at the names in the following table. There are no clues from the names as to what class of drug they belong in. This is one place where name recognition becomes very important for exam taking. You may know everything about the MAO inhibitors, but if you do not recognize that tranylcypromine belongs in that group you may well miss the question.

HETEROCYCLICS	MAO INHIBITORS	SSRIs
IMIPRAMINE	phenelzine	FLUOXETINE
DESIPRAMINE	isocarboxazid	sertraline
amitriptyline	tranylcypromine	paroxetine
nortriptyline		
doxepine		
maprotiline		

Learn what you can about each class of antidepressant and then be sure that you know the names of the drugs in each class.

HETEROCYCLICS

Most of the drugs in this class are really "tricyclics," based on their chemical structure of a three-ring core (Fig. 19-1). There are a couple of other useful antidepressants that do not have the three-ring core, but otherwise are similar in action and side effects to the tricyclic compounds. There-

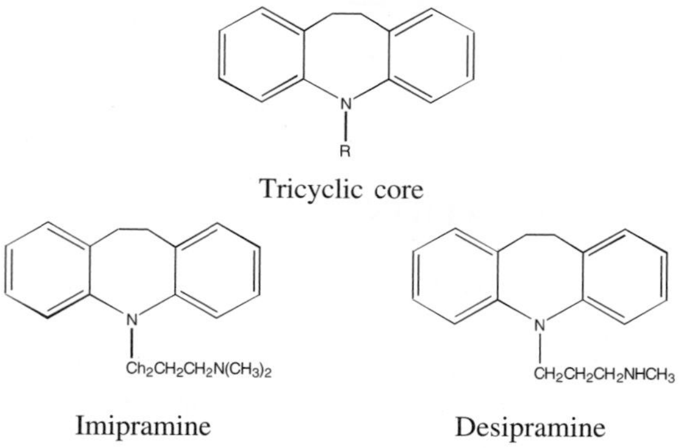

Tricyclic core

Imipramine

Desipramine

Figure 19-1
This figure shows the main structure of the tricyclic antidepressants and two examples of drugs in this class. The three rings are obvious.

fore, they should all be learned together. The drugs are all equally efficacious, but vary in potency. In addition, some patients will respond to one
drug in this class and not to another one.

Tricyclics have little effect in normal (non-depressed) people.

It takes 2 to 3 weeks of dosing with the tricyclics to see an effect on
depression.

The precise mechanism of action of the tricyclic drugs is unknown.
These drugs block the reuptake of biogenic amines, including norepinephrine and serotonin.

Heterocyclic antidepressants are:
  Potent muscarinic cholinergic antagonists
  Weak α_1 antagonists
  Weak histamine antagonists
These actions account for the major side effects of these drugs.

If you can remember these three actions of the heterocyclic antidepressants then you can also list most of the significant side effects from
your outstanding knowledge of autonomic pharmacology. The cholinergic-
blocking effect will produce dry mouth, constipation, urinary retention,
blurred vision, and so on. The α-blocking effect will produce orthostatic
hypotension and the histamine antagonism will produce sedation. Tolerance
to the anticholinergic effects does occur.

In overdose, these drugs can produce serious, life-threatening cardiac
arrhythmias, delirium, and psychosis.

SEROTONIN-SPECIFIC REUPTAKE INHIBITORS (SSRIs)

These drugs block the reuptake of serotonin. Therefore, they are referred to as *serotonin-specific reuptake inhibitors* or *selective serotonin
reuptake inhibitors*. Either name gives you the abbreviation of SSRI.

These drugs are highly selective for serotonin. Therefore, it is currently believed that the mechanism by which these drugs alleviate depression is by their blockade of the reuptake of serotonin. This may seem self-evident. If so, then it should be easy for you to remember.

SSRIs are not cholinergic antagonists or α-blockers.

This should help you keep the side effect profiles of the antidepressant classes straight.

SSRIs may cause CNS stimulation and GI upset.

The CNS stimulation by the SSRIs cause mostly agitation and nervousness. The GI upsets include nausea and vomiting.

MONOAMINE OXIDASE (MAO) INHIBITORS

Monoamine oxidase is a mitochondrial enzyme that exists in two major forms, A and B. Its major role in life is to oxidize monoamines, including norepinephrine, serotonin, and dopamine. Blocking this degradative enzyme slows the removal of transmitter.

Isocarboxazid, phenelzine, and tranylcypromine are irreversible, nonselective inhibitors of MAO-A and MAO-B. However, research suggests that the antidepressant effect of these drugs is due to inhibition of MAO-A.

The potential toxicities of the MAO inhibitors restrict their use.

MAO inhibitors can cause a FATAL hypertensive crisis.

Patients taking MAO inhibitors should not eat foods rich in tyramine or other biologically active amines. These foods include cheese, beer, and red wine. Normally, tyramine and other amines are rapidly inactivated by MAO in the gut. Individuals on MAO inhibitors are unable to inactivate the tyramine and the tyramine causes release of norepinephrine, which can lead to an increase in blood pressure and cardiac arrhythmias.

Before moving on, take a glance at the following table and see if you can rationalize the stuff there.

GROUP	CNS	BLOOD PRESSURE	ANTICHOLINERGIC EFFECTS
Heterocyclics	Sedation	↓ ↓	+++
SSRIs	Stimulation	No effect	No effect
MAOIs	Stimulation	↓, or ↑ depending on diet	+

LITHIUM

LITHIUM is the DRUG OF CHOICE for the treatment of manic-depressive illness.

Lithium can be used in the treatment of acute mania, but usually takes 1 to 3 weeks to be effective. However, chronic treatment with lithium can reduce the frequency of manic and depressive episodes and is considered a mood stabilizer. Occasionally, neuroleptics or antidepressants may be needed for breakthrough episodes of mania or depression.

The mechanism of action of lithium is not well understood, but is postulated to involve second messenger systems in the brain. Lithium is a monovalent cation that can replace Na^+ in some biological processes.

LITHIUM has a low therapeutic index and the frequency and severity of adverse reactions is directly related to the serum levels.

Frequent measurements of the serum level are routinely carried out during chronic treatment.

Lithium use is occasionally associated with hypothyroidism or nephrogenic diabetes insipidus. Both conditions are reversible upon stopping the lithium.

ANTIPSYCHOTICS OR NEUROLEPTICS

·

Class Organization

"Typical" Antipsychotics

"Atypical" Antipsychotics

·　·　·　·　·　·　·　·　·　·　·　·

CLASS ORGANIZATION

These drugs have been called neuroleptics, antischizophrenic drugs, antipsychotic drugs, and major tranquilizers. All these terms are synonymous; neuroleptic and antipsychotic are the most common. These drugs are not curative (do not eliminate the fundamental thinking disorder), but often permit the patient to function more normally. Of course, what is normal?

All of the neuroleptics are:
  α-Blockers
  Muscarinic antagonists
  Histamine antagonists
These actions produce the side effects of the drugs.

If you know which receptors these drugs block, you can predict all of the actions and side effects of these drugs. The antimuscarinic actions give dry mouth, constipation, urinary retention, blurred vision, and so on. The α-antagonism gives orthostatic hypotension and the H1 antagonism gives sedation.*

These drugs used to be organized based on their chemical structure. I do not recommend this method unless you have decided to memorize all of the structures. I recommend dividing this group of drugs into two groups: the "old," "typical" antipsychotics and the newer "atypical" drugs. The first group is much larger than the second. Name recognition here is sometimes a problem, but notice that most of the "typical" neuroleptics end in -azine.

All neuroleptics are dopamine blockers, but the typical and atypical drugs block dopamine receptors in different ways.

TYPICAL		ATYPICAL
CHLORPROMAZINE	fluphenazine	CLOZAPINE
thioridazine	trifluoperazine	loxapine
HALOPERIDOL	prochlorperazine	
thiothixene	mesoridazine	
acetophenazine	perphenazine	
chlorprothixene		

You now know the most fundamental information about the drugs in this group. You need only add a little bit more, depending on your trivia level.

"TYPICAL" ANTIPSYCHOTICS

All the drugs in this group have equal efficacy, they only vary in potency and side effect profiles.

Reminder: The typical antipsychotics block dopamine, muscarinic, cholinergic, α-adrenergic, and H_1 histaminergic receptors.

---

*Notice that these actions and side effects are very similar to the heterocyclic antidepressants.

The dopamine antagonism is believed to produce the antipsychotic effect. It also produces some endocrinological effects. Remember that dopamine inhibits prolactin release. Thus, an antagonist at the dopamine receptor will result in an increase in prolactin release. This in turn leads to lactation.

Most of the neuroleptics, EXCEPT thioridazine, have antiemetic effects that are mediated by blocking D_2 receptors of the chemoreceptor trigger zone in the medulla.

> All of these drugs produce extrapyramidal effects, including parkinsonism, akathisia, and tardive dyskinesia.

The extrapyramidal effects of these drugs are presumably due to blocking of dopamine receptors in the striatum (basal ganglia). Extrapyramidal effects include acute dystonia (spasm of the muscles of the face, tongue, neck, and back), akathisia (motor restlessness), and parkinsonism (rigidity, tremor, and shuffling gait). Because it is irreversible, one of the most worrisome extrapyramidal effects is tardive dyskinesia. Tardive dyskinesia may appear during or after prolonged therapy with any of these drugs. It involves stereotyped involuntary movements, such as lip smacking, jaw movements, and darting of the tongue. Purposeless quick movements of the limbs may also occur.

The more potent drugs produce more extrapyramidal effects. Conversely, the drugs with more anticholinergic potency have less extrapyramidal effects (Fig. 20-1). Compare this to what we know about Parkinson's disease. In Parkinson's a loss of dopamine neurons leads to a movement disorder than can be treated with anticholinergics. Here, we

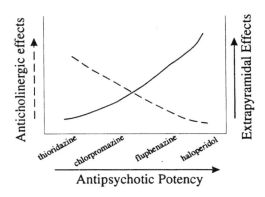

Figure 20-1
As the antipsychotics increase in potency for their antipsychotic effect, there is a trend toward a decrease in the anticholinergic side effects (dashed line) and an increase in the incidence of extrapyramidal side effects (solid line).

are using drugs to block dopamine receptors, which you may predict will lead to parkinsonism (symptoms like Parkinson's disease, but not due to a loss of neurons). Drugs with anticholinergic actions cause less extrapyramidal effects because the dopamine/acetylcholine balance in the motor systems is less affected.

"ATYPICAL" NEUROLEPTICS

CLOZAPINE causes fewer extrapyramidal effects and may not cause tardive dyskinesia.

Clozapine and other related compounds are good antipsychotic drugs that do not appear to cause extrapyramidal effects, including tardive dyskinesia. Although these drugs are still under intense investigation, there does appear to be a distinct difference in the dopamine blocking ability of these atypical drugs as compared with the typical neuroleptics. Not only do these drugs not cause extrapyramidal effects, they also do not increase prolactin levels.

CLOZAPINE has caused FATAL agranulocytosis.

Monitoring of the white cell count needs to be done on a regular basis. Since this is a life-threatening action of the drug, you may wonder why it is used at all. Clozapine has been found to be useful in patients that do not respond to the typical neuroleptics, so it is used cautiously.

Reminder: CLOZAPINE also blocks muscarinic, α_1-adrenergic, serotonin, and histamine receptors in addition to dopamine receptors.

The side effects you learned for the whole class apply to these drugs also.

> Neuroleptic malignant syndrome is a rare, potentially FATAL neurological side effect of antipsychotic medication.

Many classes do not teach about neuroleptic malignant syndrome, but since it is potentially fatal, it is worth a mention here.

Neuroleptic malignant syndrome resembles a very severe form of parkinsonism, with catatonia, autonomic instability, and stupor. It may persist for more than a week after stopping the offending drug. Since mortality is high (greater than 10 percent), immediate medical attention is required. This syndrome has occurred with all neuroleptics, but is more common with relatively high doses of the more potent agents, especially when administered parenterally.

· C H A P T E R · 2 1 ·

ANTIEPILEPTIC DRUGS
·

Class organization

Important Details About the Four Most Important Drugs

Other Drugs to Consider

· · · · · · · · · · · ·

CLASS ORGANIZATION

This class of drugs does not lend itself to the type of organization used in many other chapters. Here we need to consider the disease to be treated.

Epilepsy is a chronic disorder characterized by recurrent episodes in which the brain is subject to abnormal excessive discharges (seizures) synchronized throughout a population of neurons. The seizures themselves have been classified to assist with demographics and treatment. The table below is a simplified seizure classification scheme.

Notice that some of these seizures do not involve muscle jerking or convulsions. In particular, absence seizures are called *nonconvulsive*. Technically, this would make the name "anticonvulsants" inaccurate, but it is often used to designate this class of drugs.

Now that we have defined the types of seizures we want to treat we can

SEIZURE TYPE AND CLINICAL MANIFESTATIONS	
I. Partial (focal, local)	
A. Partial simple	Focal motor, sensory, or speech disturbance. No impairment of consciousness.
B. Partial complex	Dreamy state with automatisms. Impaired consciousness.
C. Partial seizures with secondary generalization	
II. Generalized seizures	
A. Generalized convulsive (tonic-clonic, grand mal)	Loss of consciousness, falling, rigid extension of trunk and limbs. Rhythmic contractions of arms and legs.
B. Generalized nonconvulsive (absence, petit mal)	Impaired consciousness with staring and eye blinks.

start to examine the drugs. To simplify this organization let us consider which drugs are used to treat which types of seizures.

SEIZURE TYPE	DRUGS OF CHOICE
Generalized convulsive	CARBAMAZEPINE PHENYTOIN Valproic acid*
Partial, including simple, complex and secondarily generalized	CARBAMAZEPINE PHENYTOIN
Generalized nonconvulsive	ETHOSUXIMIDE VALPROIC ACID

Often used, but debate about whether it is a primary DRUG OF CHOICE.

We have covered the drugs of choice for all of the major types of seizures using only four drugs. In addition to these four drugs, you should be aware of several others, most notably PHENOBARBITAL and PRIMIDONE.

Other facts that are easy to remember about these drugs include the following: they are *all* liver metabolized and *all,* except ethosuximide, are highly protein bound.

IMPORTANT DETAILS ABOUT THE FOUR MOST IMPORTANT DRUGS

CARBAMAZEPINE causes autoinduction of its own metabolism.

Carbamazepine is liver metabolized and over a period of several weeks induces the enzymes that metabolize carbamazepine. Therefore, an initially adequate dose gradually produces lower and lower plasma levels as the liver increases the metabolism (shortening the half-life).

Carbamazepine has been associated with granulocyte suppression and aplastic anemia.

PHENYTOIN has zero-order kinetics.

Review zero-order kinetics in Chap. 4 if this does not ring a loud bell for you. The fact that phenytoin has zero-order kinetics is particularly important because phenytoin turns into a zero-order drug right in the therapeutic range (Fig. 21-1).

PHENYTOIN causes ataxia and nystagmus at high doses. It has been associated with hirsutism, coarsening of facial features, and gingival hyperplasia.

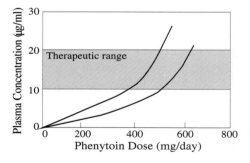

Figure 21-1
Notice that as the dose of phenytoin increases the plasma concentration does not follow in a linear fashion. The curve becomes steeper. That is where phenytoin is switching to zero-order kinetics. It is in slightly different places for different people.

Phenytoin is thought to act by blocking the sodium channel in the inactivated state. Additional details about its side effects and actions can be learned, if you are really interested.

ETHOSUXIMIDE is the DRUG OF CHOICE for absence seizures. It is associated with tummy aches, vomiting, and hiccups.

Ethosuximide is thought to act by blocking calcium channels in the thalamus.

VALPROIC ACID is associated with elevated liver enzymes, with nausea and vomiting, and with weight gain. It can also produce a tremor.

Valproic acid may produce FATAL hepatic failure. It turns out that this is most common in children under the age of 2 who are on more than one antiepileptic drug. The hepatotoxicity is not dose related; it is considered to be an idiosyncratic reaction.

OTHER DRUGS TO CONSIDER

We are getting lower down on the trivia list. If you have learned most of the material we've gone over so far, please continue. If you have had any trouble with the above material you may wish to wait and add the following details to your second or third pass through.

PHENOBARBITAL is an alternative drug for generalized convulsive and partial seizures. It is sedative. Like all barbiturates it will induce liver enzymes.

The chapter on anxiolytics and hypnotics (Chap. 18) contains additional features about the barbiturates. Use what you learned there and apply it here. Don't memorize this drug in isolation.

PRIMIDONE is metabolized to phenobarbital and phenylethylma-
lonamide (PEMA).

What you know about phenobarbital, for the most part, carries over to
primidone. There are some additional facts about primidone, if you wish to
tackle more.

Clonazepam is an alternative drug for the treatment of generalized
nonconvulsive seizures. It is a benzodiazepine and tolerance develops
to its antiepileptic effects.

The chapter on anxiolytics and hypnotics (Chap. 18) contains additional features about the benzodiazepines. Use what you learned there and
apply it here. Don't memorize this drug in isolation.

There is a fairly long list of other drugs that have been used over the
years in the treatment of epilepsy. Those of you with a particular interest in
the area can explore these drugs in more depth. You should also take a few
minutes to review the drugs used in the treatment of status epilepticus.

NARCOTICS (OPIATES)

·

Class Organization

The Actions of Morphine and, by Association, All the Other
  Agonists

Important Distinguishing Features of Some Agonists

Opioid Antagonists

Opioid Agonist–Antagonists

· · · · · · · · · · · ·

CLASS ORGANIZATION

The word narcotics (or opiates) refers to drugs that act on specific receptors in the central nervous system to reduce perception of pain. In general they do not eliminate pain, but the patient is not as bothered by the pain. They act on three major classes of receptors in the CNS, called opioid receptors and designated mu (μ), kappa (λ) and delta (δ). Most of the actions of the narcotic analgesics are mediated by the μ receptor. Some actions are mediated through the λ and δ receptors.

> Divide the narcotics into three groups:
> 1. Agonists: use morphine as prototype
> 2. Mixed agonist–antagonists
> 3. Antagonists

A partial listing of drugs in this class are included in the following table.

AGONISTS	MIXED AGONIST-ANTAGONISTS	ANTAGONISTS
MORPHINE	PENTAZOCINE	NALOXONE
MEPERIDINE	nalbuphine	NALTREXONE
CODEINE	butorphanol	
METHADONE		
HEROIN		
FENTANYL		
sufentanil		
alfentanil		
levorphanol		
hydrocodone		
dihydrocodeine		
oxycodone		
hydromorphone		
propoxyphene		
buprenorphine		
oxymorphone		

The most important drug names in this class are in capitals in the table. Notice that there are many more agonists than antagonists and that there is only one important mixed agonist–antagonist.

> Remember the names of the antagonists (naloxone and naltrexone) and the most important mixed agonist-antagonist (pentazocine). Everything else is an agonist.

Of course, that statement was somewhat simplified. Use morphine as the prototype drug in this class. The other agonists have the same general properties. They vary in things like potency and duration of action.

THE ACTIONS OF MORPHINE AND, BY ASSOCIATION, ALL THE OTHER AGONISTS

Morphine causes:
1. Analgesia
2. Respiratory depression
3. Spasm of smooth muscle of the GI and GU tract, including the biliary tract
4. Pin-point pupils

Morphine has actions in many organ systems. We will consider them one at a time. These actions are sometimes used for therapeutic purposes and sometimes are considered side effects. Therefore, learning the important actions means that you have learned both therapeutic uses and adverse effects at one time.

CNS: In most people morphine produces drowsiness and sedation in addition to the reduction in awareness of pain.

Initial doses of morphine often cause nausea, more in patients that are walking around than in bedridden patients. This is due to direct stimulation of the chemoreceptor trigger zone in the medulla oblongata and to an increase in vestibular sensitivity.

Morphine is a good cough suppressant due to a direct effect in the medulla. Morphine is not used for this purpose, but codeine (another agonist) is frequently prescribed for its cough suppressant action.

Eye: Morphine produces pupillary constriction by a direct action in the brain nucleus of the oculomotor nerve (Edinger–Westphal). This is the classic "pin-point" pupil that you will hear about in the emergency room.

Respiratory: Again through a direct action on the CNS, morphine causes respiratory depression. All phases of respiratory activity are depressed, including rate and minute volume. The hypoxic drive for breathing is also depressed.

CV: Morphine has essentially no effect on the cardiovascular system at therapeutic doses.

GI: Morphine increases the resting tone of the smooth muscle of the entire gastrointestinal tract. This results in a decrease in the movement of stomach and intestinal contents, which may lead to spasm (pain) and to constipation.

Morphine will also produce spasm of the smooth muscle of the biliary tract.

GU: Like its action on the GI tract, morphine increases the tone and produces spasm of the smooth muscle in the genitourinary tract. This can lead to urinary retention.

Withdrawal from narcotics in a dependent person consists of autonomic hyperactivity, such as diarrhea, vomiting, chills, fever, tearing, and runny nose. Tremor, abdominal cramps, and pain can be severe. As opposed to the withdrawal from sedatives, the withdrawal from narcotics is usually not life-threatening.

That was a quick summary of the most important information about morphine's actions. If you are doing well to this point, then continue on and learn some specific details of some of the agonists. If you had some trouble with the detail above, come back to the following section on another pass through the material.

IMPORTANT DISTINGUISHING FEATURES OF SOME AGONISTS

CODEINE is used for suppressing cough and for pain. It is much less potent than morphine.

HEROIN is more lipid soluble than morphine and, therefore, rapidly crosses the blood–brain barrier. It is hydrolyzed to morphine.

MEPERIDINE is less potent than morphine and less spasmogenic. It has no cough suppressive ability.

Some more detailed trivia that you may need—meperidine is also known for its use in obstetrics. Unlike morphine, meperidine produces no more respiratory depression in the fetus than in the mother.

Two relatives of meperidine (diphenoxylate and loperamide) have gained acceptance for the treatment of diarrhea. Neither is well absorbed after oral administration, so their action remains in the GI tract.

FENTANYL is 80 times more potent than morphine, but has a short duration of action. It is used by anesthesiologists.

METHADONE is a highly effective analgesic after oral administration and has a much longer duration of action than morphine.

Methadone is used in the treatment of addiction to narcotics. This is counterintuitive to some students. The knee-jerk impulse is to think of treating addicts with an antagonist. This, however, would put them into immediate and frightening withdrawal. The idea is to replace the addict's heroin with an orally active agonist with a long duration of action. This reduces the drug craving and prevents the withdrawal. Do not be tempted to think of methadone as an antagonist.

Before we leave the agonists, you should be aware that the opiates are often used in combination with the non-opiate analgesics (aspirin and acetaminophen). Since these different classes of drugs effect pain pathways by different mechanisms, the combinations have proven to be effective in producing analgesia with fewer side effects.

OPIOID ANTAGONISTS

Opioid antagonists have no effect when administered alone. When given after a dose of agonist, they promptly reverse all of the actions of the agonist.

This is basically the definition of antagonist from general principles.

NALOXONE is the DRUG OF CHOICE for narcotic overdose.

OPIOID AGONIST–ANTAGONISTS

The concept of a mixed agonist–antagonist is confusing to many students. Unlike antagonists, these compounds have an action when given alone. That's why they are called agonists. When they are administered after a dose of agonist, they will reverse most of the actions of the agonist. Thus they are also antagonistic. This leads to the classification as mixed agonist–antagonists.

PENTAZOCINE produces effects that are qualitatively similar to morphine.

Pentazocine will cause acute withdrawal in patients who have received regular doses of morphine or other agonist.

GENERAL ANESTHETICS

·

Class Organization

Uptake and Distribution of Inhalational Anesthetics

Elimination of Inhalational Anesthetics

Potency of General Anesthetics

Specific Gases and Volatile Liquids

Specific Intravenous Agents

· · · · · · · · · · · ·

CLASS ORGANIZATION

The state of general anesthesia is a drug-induced absence of perception of all sensations. Depths of anesthesia appropriate for surgical procedures can be achieved with a wide variety of drugs. General anesthetics are administered primarily by inhalation and intravenous injection. These routes of administration allow control of the dosage and time course of action.

For these drugs, understanding the principles of uptake, distribution and elimination are the major focus, particularly for the inhaled anesthetics. The mechanism of action of most of the anesthetics is unknown. You should be able to recognize the names of the general anesthetics and know a few specific facts (Fig. 23-1).

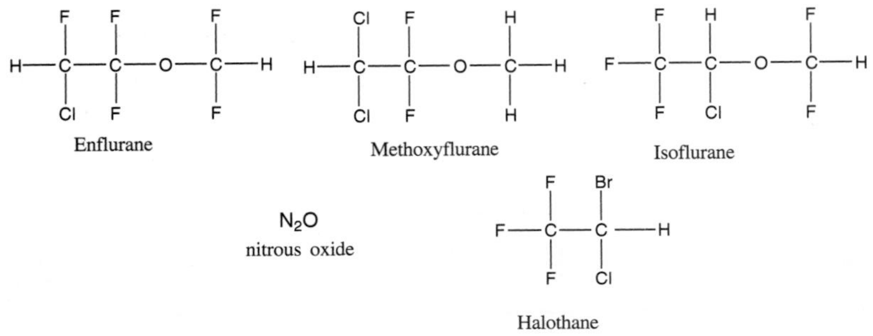

Figure 23-1
Structures of some of the inhalational drugs. Notice the very simple structures and the presence of fluoride.

INHALED	INTRAVENOUS
HALOTHANE	THIOPENTAL
ENFLURANE	PROPOFOL
ISOFLURANE	ketamine
NITROUS OXIDE	etomidate
methoxyflurane	

UPTAKE AND DISTRIBUTION OF INHALATIONAL ANESTHETICS

The tension of a gas in a mixture is proportional to its concentration. Therefore, the terms *tension* and *concentration* are often used interchangeably. The term *partial pressure* is also used interchangeably with tension.

When a constant tension (concentration) of anesthetic gas is inhaled, the tension (concentration) in arterial blood approaches that of the agent in the inspired mixture. The tension (concentration) in the brain is always approaching the tension (concentration) in arterial blood.

The level of general anesthesia is dependent on the concentration of anesthetic in the brain.

> The solubility of an agent is expressed as the blood:gas partition coefficient.

The blood:gas partition coefficient represents the ratio of anesthetic concentration in blood to the concentration in the gas phase. The blood:gas coefficient is high for very soluble agents and low for relatively insoluble anesthetics, such as nitrous oxide.

> The more soluble an anesthetic is in blood, the more of it must be dissolved in blood to raise its partial pressure in the blood.

The potential reservoir for relatively soluble gases is large and will be filled more slowly. Therefore, for soluble gases the rate at which the tension (partial pressure) in the arterial blood approaches the inspired partial pressure is slow. Also, the rate at which the brain partial pressure approaches the arterial partial pressure is slow. The opposite is true for more insoluble anesthetics.

> The speed of onset of anesthesia is inversely related to the solubility of the gas in blood.
> More soluble: high blood:gas partition coefficient = slower onset
> Less soluble: low blood:gas partition coefficient = faster onset

Onset of anesthesia is also related to pulmonary ventilation, rate of pulmonary blood flow, tissue blood flow, and solubility of the gas in the tissues.

ELIMINATION OF INHALATIONAL ANESTHETICS

> Elimination of anesthetics is influenced by pulmonary ventilation, blood flow, and solubility of the gas.

The major factors that affect the rate of elimination of the anesthetics are the same factors that are important in the uptake phase. That makes these principles easy to remember.

Most of the inhaled anesthetics are eliminated unchanged in the exhaled gas. A small percentage of the anesthetics are metabolized in the liver. It has been suggested that the production of a toxic metabolite may be responsible for most of the hepatic and renal toxicities observed with these agents. One example of this is methoxyflurane. It has been associated with renal failure as a result of toxic amounts of fluoride ions produced when the drug is metabolized. More details on this are available in your local textbook.

POTENCY OF GENERAL ANESTHETICS

Anesthesiologists have accepted a measure of potency for the inhalational anesthetics known as MAC.

Minimum alveolar concentration (MAC) is defined as the alveolar concentration at 1 atmosphere that produces immobility in 50 percent of patients exposed to a noxious stimulus.

The MAC is usually expressed as the percentage of gas in the mixture required to achieve immobility in 50 percent of patients exposed to a painful stimulus. The alveolar concentration is used for this definition because the concentration in the lung can be easily and accurately measured. The real concentration that we would want to know is the brain concentration. It is not so easy to measure brain levels, but we know that brain levels are directly correlated to alveolar levels. So, the MAC is a good approximation of brain levels.

SPECIFIC GASES AND VOLATILE LIQUIDS

Each of these drugs has a whole range of effects on the lungs, heart, and circulation. It is probably advisable to read through a detailed description of these effects and pick out some trends to memorize. See, for example, the table below that compares some features of the more common inhalational agents. Notice that nitrous oxide stands out as being different.

ANES-THETIC	ANAL-GESIA	BLOOD PRESSURE	RESPIRATION	MUSCLE RELAXATION	MAC (%)
Halothane	2+	↓	↓ ↓	+	0.77
Enflurane	2+	↓	↓ ↓	2+	1.68
Isoflurane	2+	↓	↓ ↓	2+	1.15
Nitrous oxide	4+	Little effect	Little effect	none	105

NITROUS OXIDE is a relatively insoluble gas with a MAC of about 105 percent, which has little effect on blood pressure or respiration. Does produce analgesia.

The low solubility means that onset of anesthesia with nitrous oxide is very fast. The MAC indicates that nitrous oxide has very low potency. So low in fact, that more than 100 percent of the inspired gas needs to be nitrous oxide to produce immobility in 50 percent of patients exposed to a noxious stimulus. That's why nitrous oxide is used in combination with other agents.

HALOTHANE causes myocardial depression and may produce FA-TAL hepatitis.

The hepatitis is a rare occurrence, but is probably why halothane is not used as much these days as in yesteryear. Halothane is also reported to sensitize the myocardium to catecholamines, increasing the likelihood of cardiac arrhythmias.

ISOFLURANE is metabolized much less than halothane or enflu-rane. Therefore, it has potentially less hepatotoxicity.

SPECIFIC INTRAVENOUS AGENTS

The majority of intravenous drugs used to induce anesthesia are slowly metabolized and excreted, and depend on redistribution to terminate their pharmacological effects.

Ultra-short-acting barbiturates are commonly used to induce anesthesia.

The barbiturates are covered in detail in Chap. 18. Thiopental, thiamylal, and methohexital are useful for anesthesia. It is just a matter of adding what you already know about barbiturates to these names and associating them with anesthesia. These drugs do *not* produce analgesia.

Benzodiazepines such as diazepam, lorazepam, and midazolam have found use as anesthetic agents.

The benzodiazepines are covered in detail in Chap. 18. As with the barbiturates, these drugs do *not* cause analgesia.

Ketamine causes dissociative anesthesia.

This is a bit more trivial, but interesting if you have the time and energy to study its effects.

PROPOFOL and etomidate are two other drugs use intravenously to produce general anesthesia.

On first pass you should recognize these names and know that they are general anesthetics. On the second pass, you should try to add some details about analgesia and cardiovascular effects.

LOCAL ANESTHETICS

·

Class Organization

Mechanism of Action

Special Features about Individual Agents

·   ·   ·   ·   ·   ·   ·   ·   ·   ·   ·   ·

CLASS ORGANIZATION

These drugs are applied locally and block nerve conduction. Peripheral nerve functions are not affected equally. Loss of sympathetic function occurs first, followed by loss of pin-prick sensation, touch and temperature, and, lastly, motor function. The effect of local anesthetics is reversible: their use is followed by complete recovery of nerve function with no evidence of structural damage.

All the local anesthetics consist of a hydrophilic amino group linked through a connecting group of variable length to a lipophilic aromatic portion (benzene ring) (Fig. 24-1). Both the potency and toxicity of the local anesthetics increase as the connecting group becomes longer. In the intermediate chain, there is either an ester linkage or an amide linkage.

The commonly used local anesthetics can be classified as esters or amides based on the linkage in this intermediate chain. The amide local anesthetics are chemically stable in vivo, while the esters are rapidly hydrolyzed by plasma cholinesterase. One interesting trivial fact is that metabo-

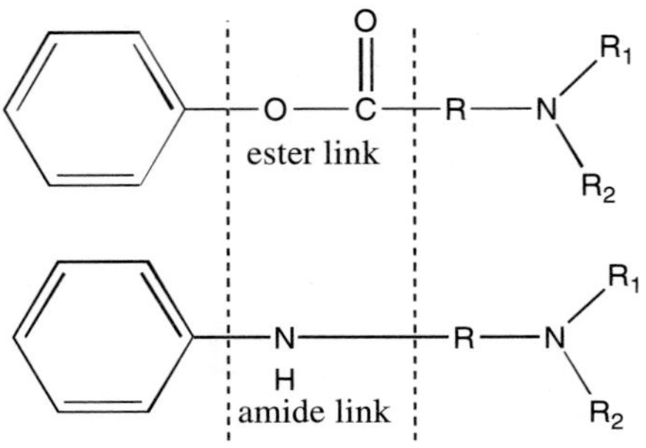

Figure 24-1
Main structures for the ester
and amide local anesthetics.

lism of the ester local anesthetics leads to formation of *para*-aminobenzoic
acid (PABA), which is known to be allergenic.

ESTERS	AMIDES
COCAINE	LIDOCAINE
benzocaine	bupivacaine
chlorprocaine	etidocaine
PROCAINE	mepivacaine
tetracaine	prilocaine
	ropivacaine

The *-caine* ending on each of these drugs tells you that they are local
anesthetics, but the names don't really give any clues about the ester versus
amide linkage.

Adverse effects of the local anesthetics result from systemic absorption of toxic amounts of the drugs.

DEATH can occur from respiratory failure secondary to medullary
depression or from hypotension and cardiovascular collapse.

MECHANISM OF ACTION

Local anesthetics block the sodium channel in the nerve membrane.

Application of a local anesthetic will inhibit the inward movement of Na^+ ions. This will result in elevation of the threshold for electrical excitation, reduction in the rate of rise of the action potential, and slowing of the propagation of the impulse. At high enough concentrations the local anesthetics will completely block conduction of impulses down the nerve.

For those of you interested in this area, there is a fascinating story relating pH to ionization of the local anesthetics to drug action. For details, see you favorite textbook.

SPECIAL FEATURES ABOUT INDIVIDUAL AGENTS

> LIDOCAINE is a local anesthetic used in the treatment of cardiac arrhythmias.

> COCAINE is better known as a drug of abuse, but it is an effective local anesthetic.

CHEMOTHERAPEUTIC AGENTS

·

· C H A P T E R · 2 5 ·

INTRODUCTION TO CHEMOTHERAPY

·

Approach to the Antimicrobials

General Principles of Therapy

Definitions

Big Concepts to Understand

Classification of Antimicrobials

· · · · · · · · · · · ·

APPROACH TO THE ANTIMICROBIALS

Students often have a very difficult time with the antibiotics, not because of any difficult concepts, but because of the large number of drugs. It is also overwhelming to try to memorize the bugs that are sensitive to each drug.

So . . . try this approach.

First, make absolutely sure that you understand the general principles of therapy and some definitions. We will go over these in this chapter.

Second, be aware of the classes of antibiotics and the mechanism of action for the class. Note any features that are common to *all* drugs in the class.

Third, learn the particular adverse effects or special features of administration for the drugs in the class. Do any of the drugs cause potentially FATAL side effects?

Fourth, learn the broad categories of bacterial spectrum and whether any of the drugs in the class are the DRUG OF CHOICE for the treatment of a particular bug. For example, are the drugs good against all gram-positive, but none of the gram-negative? It may be useful to do a quick review of the bacteria at this point. Can you quickly say which bugs are the gram-positive and which are the gram-negative? It will really help when you are trying to learn the antibiotics.

This looks like a long list of things to learn, but it is really quite manageable. Remember not to get too bogged down in trying to remember the second-line drugs for treatment of certain bugs, which drug to use in case of allergies, and so on. This can be added on later to a base of knowledge that is developed now.

GENERAL PRINCIPLES OF THERAPY

> To be a useful antibiotic, a compound should inhibit the growth of bacteria without harming the human host.

This should be self-evident, but it is the basis for understanding most of the mechanisms of action of these drugs. The compound should affect some aspect of bacteria that is not present in mammalian cells. We'll come back to that later.

> The drug should penetrate body tissues in order to reach the bacteria.

This again should be self-evident. (I told you this stuff is not hard.) Again, this is the basis for needing to know if a drug is orally absorbed and whether it will cross the blood–brain barrier. If the patient has a GI infection, then give a drug orally that is not absorbed. The bug gets treated and the patient has few side effects. The drugs that are used to treat meningitis are ones that cross the blood–brain barrier. The drug that is extremely effective against *Hemophilus influenza* does no good for the patient if the drug cannot reach the bugs.

DEFINITIONS

Spectrum, as in narrow, broad and extended spectrum, is a term used to convey an impression of the range of bacteria that a drug will treat.

Drugs are designated narrow spectrum if they are only effective against one class of bacteria. They are designated broad spectrum if they are effective against a range of bacteria. If a narrow spectrum agent is modified chemically (as in adding a new side chain), and the new compound is effective against more bugs than the parent compound, then the new drug is said to have an extended spectrum. Easy enough!

Bacteriostatic versus bactericidal.

Books often make a big deal about knowing whether a drug will arrest the growth and replication of a bacteria (static) or whether a drug will actually kill the bacteria (cidal). If a drug is bacteriostatic, the patients immune system must complete the task of clearing the body of the invaders. Don't focus too much time on this early on. I will point out some of the easy ones to remember as we go through the drugs. Later if you have time and energy learn a few more.

BIG CONCEPTS TO UNDERSTAND

Resistance of a bacteria to an antibiotic can occur by mutation, adaptation, or gene transfer.

The whole area of bacterial resistance has received much attention lately and appropriately so. Many of the bacteria are becoming resistant to the available drugs. Students need to have some idea of the mechanisms of bacterial resistance.

Bacteria undergo spontaneous *mutation* at a frequency of about 1 in 10 cells. The mutation may make the bacteria resistant to the antibiotic, or it may not.

Adaptation can take several routes. The bacteria may alter the uptake of the drug by changes in the lipopolysaccharide coat. Or, a bacteria may improve a transport system that removes the drug from the cell. The bacteria may increase metabolism through a pathway that bypasses the effect of the antibiotic.

Gene transfer occurs through plasmids and transposons. Plasmids are extrachromosomal genetic elements (pieces of RNA or DNA that are not part of chromosomes). These may code for enzymes that inactivate antimicrobials. The plasmids are transferred from bacteria to bacteria by conjugation and transduction. Transposons are segments of genetic material with insertion sequences. They get incorporated into the genetic makeup of the bacteria and also can code for enzymes that inactivate the antimicrobials.

Adverse effects can be allergic, toxic, idiosyncratic, or related to changes in the normal body flora.

There are general categories for the adverse effects of antibiotics. The first three (allergic, toxic, and idiosyncratic) are categories that are true for all drugs. The last (changes in normal body flora) is unique to antibiotics.

Just as a reminder. Idiosyncratic reactions are reactions that are not related to immune responses or known drug properties. The hemolysis in glucose-6-phosphate dehydrogenase (G-6-PD) deficient patients after treatment with sulfonamides, and the peripheral neuropathy after isoniazid in genetically slow acetylators, are examples of idiosyncratic reactions.

Alterations in the normal body flora generally refers to the gastrointestinal tract (GI tract). Normally, the gut is host to friendly bacteria that help in the digestion of stuff we eat. If an antimicrobial agent is given orally, it may kill the friendly bacteria. Other bacteria that are resistant to the antimicrobial can overgrow and repopulate the GI tract. This secondary infection is sometimes called a *superinfection.* The most common example is the overgrowth of *Clostridium difficile.* It produces a toxin that causes a disorder called *pseudomembranous colitis.* As you read in your textbook, you will probably see comments about the incidence of colitis after use of antibiotic X or antibiotic Y.

Possible site of drug action:
Protein synthesis
Cell membrane integrity
Cell wall synthesis
Nucleic acid structure and function
Production of a key metabolite

Here we are looking for sites of action that are specific for bacteria. The cell wall is an obvious place to start. Mammalian cells don't have a cell wall. Protein synthesis is another place to look since bacteria have different ribosomal units than mammalian cells. We'll come back to these mechanisms in more detail later.

Combinations of antimicrobial agents can take advantage of the mechanisms of action to get a synergistic effect.

The area of drug combinations is where an understanding of the mechanisms of action of the antimicrobials becomes important. You can combine agents with different sites of action.

For example, combine a protein synthesis inhibitor (these are static, i.e., they stop cell growth) with a drug that affects cell wall synthesis (requires cell to be dividing to have an action). Does this combination make sense?*

Another example: Two drugs both inhibit production of a key metabolic product, but at two different sites in the metabolic pathway. Does this combination make sense?†

Another example: The combination of a cell wall synthesis inhibitor and a drug that needs to act intracellularly. Does this combination make sense?‡

*This combination does not make sense. The protein synthesis inhibitor will stop cell growth and prevent cell division so that the second drug will have no effect (except possible side effects).

†This combination is useful. The two drugs (trimethoprim and sulfamethoxazole) inhibit the synthesis of folic acid at different steps in the pathway. They, in a sense, help each other out.

‡This combination is extremely useful. This is the combination of penicillins and aminoglycosides. The penicillins alter the cell wall and enhances the penetration of the aminoglycoside.

Culture and sensitivity testing will determine the MIC for the bacteria.

The best way to determine the proper antimicrobial agent for the patient is to culture and identify the organism. The lab can then run a test for sensitivity of the organism to a series of antimicrobials. They can determine the minimum inhibitory concentration (MIC), which is the lowest concentration of the drug that will inhibit growth of the organism. The drug to which the bug is most sensitive will have the lowest MIC. Culture and sensitivity (C and S) testing is extremely useful in the selection of the best antimicrobial agent to use, but can take several days depending on the growth rate of the organism.

Now . . . on to the drugs.

CLASSIFICATION OF ANTIMICROBIALS

Inhibitors of cell wall synthesis
    β-Lactams
        penicillins
        cephalosporins
        imipenem
        aztreonam
    polypeptides
        vancomycin
        bacitracin
Folate antagonists
    sulfonamides and trimethoprim
Protein synthesis inhibitors
    tetracyclines
    aminoglycosides
    erythromycin
    chloramphenicol
    clindamycin
Quinolones and other drugs
    quinolones
    urinary tract antiseptics

Notice how your book organizes these drugs. Some books focus more on structure and others more on mechanisms. Don't let this confuse you.

INHIBITORS OF CELL WALL SYNTHESIS

•

Features Common to All of the Drugs in This Group

β-Lactams

Polypeptides

• • • • • • • • • • • •

FEATURES COMMON TO *ALL* OF THE DRUGS IN THIS GROUP

All of the cell wall inhibitors are bactericidal.

All of these drugs kill bacteria by preventing the synthesis or repair of the cell wall. The cell wall protects the bacteria and prevents them from exploding.

> The penicillins, cephalosporins, vancomycin, imipenem, and aztreonam all work by inhibiting the synthesis of the bacterial cell wall.

You probably guessed this from the title of the chapter. However, this is a really key point. If you can remember this you are well on your way.

The final step in the synthesis of the bacterial cell wall is a cross-linking of adjacent peptidoglycan strands by a process called *transpeptidation*. The penicillins and cephalosporins are structurally similar to the terminal portion of the peptidoglycan strands and can compete for and bind to the enzymes that catalyze the transpeptidation and cross-linking. These enzymes are called penicillin-binding proteins (PBP). Interference with these enzymes results in the formation of a structurally weakened cell wall, odd shaped bacteria, and ultimately death.

Now, let us divide the cell wall synthesis inhibitors into two groups based on chemical structure: β-lactams and polypeptides.

β-LACTAMS

> *All* of the drugs in this group contain a β-lactam ring in their structure.

Normally, we do not worry too much about the structures of drugs, but in this case we make an important exception. These drugs are often referred to as the β-lactam group. This is because they all have a β-lactam ring in their chemical structure and it is this β-lactam ring that makes them effective antimicrobials.

> Inactivation of the β-lactam antibiotics is by an enzyme in the bacteria that opens the β-lactam ring.

Some bacteria contain an enzyme, called β-lactamase, that can open the β-lactam ring (Fig. 26-1). This leads to inactivation of the antibiotic. The most common mode of drug resistance is plasmid transfer of genetic code for the β-lactamase enzyme. There is a β-lactamase specific for the

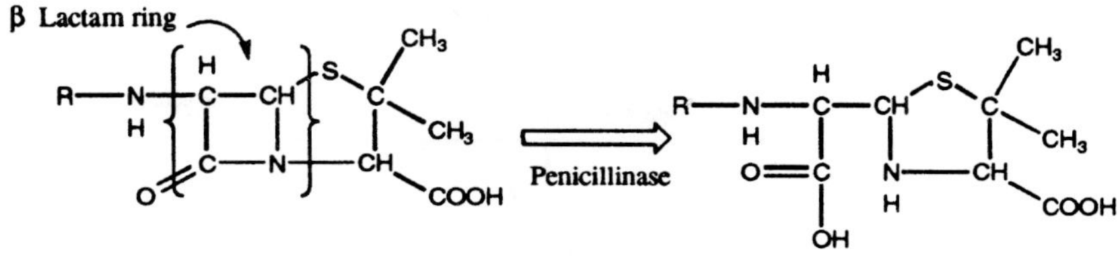

Figure 26-1
Here is shown the β-lactam ring and its opening by penicillinase.

penicillins (it is called *penicillinase*) and a β-lactamase specific for the cephalosporins (it is called *cephalosporinase*). Easy enough??

The inactivation of these drugs by the β-lactamases can be dealt with by two approaches.
1. Give a β-lactamase inhibitor at the same time.
2. Make chemical modifications in the structure of the drug to make it more resistant to inactivation.

Inactivation of these drugs by β-lactamases is a major problem and has been the focus of intense work. As you will see, one approach has been to chemically modify the structure of the compounds to make the β-lactam ring more difficult for the enzyme to open.

CLAVULANIC ACID and SULBACTAM are β-lactamase inhibitors that are given together with the β-lactam drugs to increase their effectiveness.

The other way to increase the effectiveness of the β-lactam antibiotics is to give a β-lactamase inhibitor at the same time. The most commonly used ones are clavulinic acid and sulbactam. You may also run across tazobactam.

You now know a heck of a lot about the penicillins and cephalosporins and we haven't even listed them yet. See, this is really not too difficult.

PENICILLINS

Most books divide the penicillins into three or four groups. The naturally-occurring ones are those that are made by the mold. The rest are

chemical modifications of these original penicillins, which try to improve the
bacterial spectrum and improve resistance to the penicillinase (β-lactamase).

Natural	
PENICILLIN G	Narrow spectrum (gram-positive), penicil-
PENICILLIN V	linase
benzathine pen G	sensitive
Penicillinase-resistant	
METHICILLIN	Narrow spectrum (gram-positive), synthe-
nafcillin	sized to be penicillinase-resistant
oxacillin	
cloxacillin	
dicloxacillin	
Aminopenicillins	
AMPICILLIN	Broad spectrum (some gram-negative also),
AMOXICILLIN	penicillinase-sensitive
Extended spectrum	
carbenicillin	Active against Pseudomonas, relatively inef-
ticarcillin	fective against gram-positives
mezlocillin	
azlocillin	
piperacillin	

   First of all notice that the penicillins are easy to identify by the *-cillin*
ending. The first group contains the G and V penicillins. The second group
contains the three *oxa*cillins. The third group start with *am-* for amino
group. Except for methicillin and nafcillin, the rest are in the last group.
See this is really not too hard. Keep them categorized and remember the
general outline for the spectrum and you're doing great!
   The oral absorption of the penicillins is poor, however, there are excep-
tions. If you have time and energy, you can learn the orally active ones.
Most only cross the blood–brain barrier if it is inflamed. If you have time,
add the ones that can be used in meningitis.

Penicillins are excreted by tubular secretion that can be blocked by probenecid.

   The penicillins are, for the most part, excreted by active tubular secretion. Blocking tubular excretion is a relatively simple way to prolong the

action of the drug. Probenecid can be administered along with the penicillins and it blocks the tubular secretion.

The most important adverse effect of penicillins as a group is the hypersensitivity reaction. It can be FATAL.

All penicillins can give rise to allergic reactions. These reactions have been divided into three types: immediate, accelerated, and late. The immediate is the most severe.

The immediate reaction occurs within 20 minutes after parenteral administration and consists of apprehension, itching (pruritus), paresthesia (numbness and tingling), wheezing, choking, fever, edema, and generalized urticaria (hives). It can lead to hypotension, shock, loss of consciousness, and death.

The accelerated reaction appears 1 to 72 hours after drug administration and it consists mainly of urticaria (hives).

The late reaction is more common with the semisynthetics and appears 72 hours to several weeks after drug administration. It consists mainly of skin rashes.

The immediate hypersensitivity reaction to penicillin appears to be mediated by IgE antibodies to the minor determinants.

Penicillins are metabolized to penicilloyl derivatives. These derivatives can act as haptens and combine with carrier proteins to form what is called the major determinant of penicillin allergy. Other breakdown products can also act as haptens and are known as the minor determinants. The immediate allergic reaction is thought to be mediated by IgE antibodies to the minor determinants and the accelerated and late reactions mediated by antibodies to the major determinants.

This can be difficult to remember because of the names that were given to the breakdown products. Just remember that the *minor* determinants cause the *major* reaction (the potentially FATAL immediate reaction).

How are you doing?? I hope that the penicillins don't seem too bad now. Are you ready to tackle the cephalosporins?

Trivial fact bonus: All patients with mononucleosis treated with ampicillin get a rash.

CEPHALOSPORINS

These are classified into "generations." It is impossible to learn all these names, so focus on the differences in the "generations" and try to learn three names in each generation. I have listed only three of the more common ones.

FIRST GENERATION	SECOND GENERATION	THIRD GENERATION
Narrow specrum similar to broad spectrum penicillins, sensitive to β-lactamases	Increased activity towards gram-negative, increased stability	Even broader spectrum and more stability to β-lactamases
CEPHALEXIN CEFAZOLIN	CEFACLOR CEFOXITIN CEFAMANDOLE	CEFOTAXIME CEFTRIAXONE CEFTAZIDINE

Believe it or not, this is most of what you need to know! Add a few facts about absorption, distribution, and elimination and you're golden.

Some of these drugs can be given orally (such as cephalexin and cefaclor). You can learn these if you want to try.

> In general, the third generation cephalosporins (and some second) penetrate the CNS and can be used to treat meningitis.

The third generation cephalosporins are used extensively in the treatment and prophylaxis of infections in hospitalized patients.

The cephalosporins are largely eliminated by tubular secretion (like the penicillins), and are relatively nontoxic. A few facts to consider learning:

1. There is some cross-allergy with penicillins.
2. Some cephalosporins have anti–vitamin K effects (bleeding).
3. Some cephalosporins can cause a disulfiram-like reaction because they block alcohol oxidation and acetaldehyde accumulates.

IMIPENEM

This is a relatively new β-lactam. It has a low molecular weight and easily penetrates cells. Imipenem is only administered IV.

> IMIPENEM with CILASTATIN is the broadest spectrum β-lactam antibiotic that is currently available.

Imipenem is the antibiotic. It is hydrolyzed by a renal dipeptidase on the luminal brush border of proximal tubular epithelium (i.e., in the kidney) to a somewhat toxic metabolite that is inactive as an antimicrobial. Cilastatin inhibits the renal dipeptidase. Therefore, the two compounds are always administered together.

MONOBACTAMS/AZTREONAM

The term *monobactam* refers to the chemical structure of this new class of β-lactams. The only one currently available is aztreonam.

> AZTREONAM is an excellent drug for gram-negatives, including *Pseudomonas*, but is ineffective against gram-positives.

This drug is an example of a narrow-spectrum drug. It has a kind of unusual spectrum, especially compared with the other β-lactams, so it is a good idea to file this one away in the old memory banks.

POLYPEPTIDES

These last two cell wall synthesis inhibitors are not β-lactam compounds, but are polypeptides.

VANCOMYCIN

Vancomycin and it's newest relative, teicoplanin, are glycopeptides that inhibit cell wall synthesis by preventing polymerization of the linear peptidoglycans.

VANCOMYCIN is the DRUG OF CHOICE for the treatment of *C. difficile.*

Vancomycin has a very narrow spectrum of action in that it is *only* effective against the gram-positive organisms. It is very poorly absorbed orally, which leads us to one of its special uses. Pseudomembranous colitis is caused by *Clostridium difficile,* which is sensitive to vancomycin. Give vancomycin orally and it kills the organism and then is not absorbed orally, so—behold—no toxicity.

VANCOMYCIN can cause ototoxicity.

Vancomycin can cause a dose-related ototoxicity that produces tinnitus (ringing), high-tone deafness, hearing loss, and possible deafness. This is serious enough to commit to memory.

Rapid IV infusion can cause "red man" or "red neck" syndrome. This is characterized by chills, fever, and rash, and is due to increased levels of histamine.

BACITRACIN

This is the last of the cell wall inhibitors. It also is not a β-lactam compound, but is a mixture of polypeptides.

Bacitracin is a mixture of polypeptides that inhibit cell wall synthesis. It is used topically.

Bacitracin binds to a lipid carrier that transports cell wall precursors to the growing cell wall. Therefore, it can be classified as a cell wall synthesis inhibitor.

Bacitracin has serious nephrotoxicity, so it is only used topically.

PROTEIN SYNTHESIS INHIBITORS

·

General Features of the Protein Synthesis Inhibitors

Aminoglycosides

Tetracyclines

Macrolides

Chloramphenicol

Clindamycin

·　·　·　·　·　·　·　·　·　·　·　·　·

GENERAL FEATURES OF THE PROTEIN
SYNTHESIS INHIBITORS

The protein synthesis inhibitors bind to either the 30S or 50S ribosomal subunit and interfere with the transcription of mRNA into protein.

Bacterial ribosomal subunits are different from mammalian ones. This accounts for the selectivity of the drugs for bacteria.

Classes of protein synthesis inhibitors include:

aminoglycosides: cidal, 30S
tetracyclines: 30S
macrolides/erythromycin: 50S
chloramphenicol: 50S
clindamycin: 50S

These class names are related to the chemical structure of the compounds in each group. *Only* the aminoglycosides are cidal; the rest are static. This is further down on the trivia list, but shouldn't be too hard to remember.

Resistance to these drugs is related to decreased uptake of the drugs or to altered ribosomal subunits.

Notice that these drugs require binding to an intracellular protein (ribosomal subunit). Therefore, the drugs need to get into the cell. A major route of resistance for the bacteria is to block the movement of the drugs into the cell.

AMINOGLYCOSIDES

amikacin   TOBRAMYCIN
GENTAMICIN   kanamycin
neomycin   streptomycin
netilmicin

Notice that they all end in *-mycin* or *-micin,* except amikacin. However, the drug-naming people wanted to throw you a curve ball here. Notice that the drug clindamycin and all the macrolides (erythromycin, clarithromycin, and so on) also end in *-mycin.* So take a moment and compare the lists of names. Be sure that you can recognize which class a particular name fits in.

> The aminoglycosides bind to the 30S ribosomal subunit.

Some books and courses make a point to have the students know the specific ribosomal subunit to which the class of drugs bind. However, this is not of *primary* importance. If you already know it, try not to forget it. If you are struggling with the antimicrobials at this point, save this fact for later.

> Aminoglycosides are poorly absorbed from the GI tract and are polar molecules.

Most aminoglycosides must be administered parenterally. They are highly polar compounds and are relatively insoluble in fat. They do not readily penetrate most cells without help from penicillins or a transport system.

Remember the synergism between penicillins and aminoglycosides that was mentioned in the introduction to chemotherapy. The penicillins cause cell wall abnormalities that allow the aminoglycosides to get into the bacteria.

> The aminoglycosides are broad spectrum antimicrobials. However, anaerobic bacteria are generally resistant.

Some bacteria use an oxygen-dependent transport system to bring the aminoglycosides into the cell. The anaerobes (nonoxygen-based metabolism) do not have this system. Therefore, they are generally resistant to the aminoglycosides.

> Aminoglycosides have ototoxicity, nephrotoxicity, and neuromuscular toxicity.

The margin of safety with these drug is small. This means that the toxic concentration is only slightly above the therapeutic concentration.

The ototoxicity can be both cochlear (auditory) and vestibular. The symptoms include tinnitus (ringing), deafness, vertigo or unsteadiness of gait, and high-frequency hearing loss. The cochlear toxicity is due to selective destruction of the outer hair cells in the organ of Corti.

The nephrotoxicity is related to the rapid uptake of the drug by proximal tubular cells. The proximal tubular cells are then killed. Acute nephrotoxicity is reversible.

The neurotoxicity is due to the blockade of presynaptic release of acetylcholine at the neuromuscular junction. There is also some postsynaptic blockade as well. This leads to weakness and can lead to respiratory depression.

TETRACYCLINES

TETRACYCLINE	doxycycline
demeclocycline	minocycline
chlortetracycline	oxytetracycline

These drug names are easy to recognize, because they all end in -*cycline*.

The tetracyclines also bind to the 30S ribosomal subunit, but are bacteriostatic. Similar to the aminoglycosides, the tetracyclines accumulate in the cytoplasm by an energy-dependent transport system. This transport system is not present in mammalian cells. Resistance is due to an inability of the bacteria to accumulate drug.

Tetracyclines are broad spectrum antibiotics.

Tetracyclines are useful in the treatment of gram-positive and gram-negative facultative organisms and anaerobes.

Tetracyclines have found use in the treatment of rickettsial diseases (Rocky Mountain Spotted Fever), chlamydial diseases, cholera, Lyme disease (spirochetes), and in *Mycoplasma* pneumonia.

Notice that tetracyclines are useful in the treatment of some of the "odd-ball" diseases, particularly the rickettsia and spirochetes.

Food impairs the absorption of the tetracyclines.

Except for doxycycline and minocycline, food impairs the absorption of the tetracyclines. The tetracyclines will form insoluble chelates with calcium, magnesium, and other metals. The use of antacids when taking tetracyclines is therefore unadvised.

Tetracyclines are associated with staining of the teeth, retardation of bone growth, and with photosensitivity.

The major side effects of the tetracyclines are related to its incorporation into teeth and bone. It causes the teeth to be discolored and can retard bone growth. For these reasons it is not recommended for use in children or pregnant women. There is an increased incidence of an abnormal sunburn reaction in people taking tetracyclines.

MACROLIDES

Again, this name comes from the structure of the drugs in this class. The macrolides bind to the 50S subunit of the bacterial ribosome.

ERYTHROMYCIN   clarithromycin
azithromycin

Again, these names are easy to recognize because they all end in -*romycin,* mostly -*thromycin.* Thus, they should be readily distinguishable from the aminoglycoside -*mycins.*

Erythromycin and its friends are generally well absorbed orally, although food can interfere. They are excreted in the bile.

Erythromycin and friends are of particular use in the treatment of *Mycoplasma* pneumonia, Legionnaire's disease, chlamydial infections, diphtheria, and pertussis.

Books vary somewhat on their designation of erythromycin as the DRUG OF CHOICE for some of these diseases. Check with your book or class notes and highlight those that you need to know. Notice that these are more of the "odd-ball" infections. Compare and contrast the tetracyclines and erythromycin. If you can't remember and someone asks the DRUG OF CHOICE for rickettsia or Legionnaire's, guess tetracycline or erythromycin. Better yet learn these few "odd-ones." One mnemonic that is sometimes used to remember the bugs for which erythromycin is the drug of choice is: Legionnaires Camp on My Border, legionella campylobacter mycoplasma bordatella.

The macrolides have few serious side effects. None that deserve a box of its own. GI upset is common, but you would have guessed that one—right? (wouldn't you??) These drugs can induce liver microsomal enzymes.

CHLORAMPHENICOL

Chloramphenicol stands in a class by itself. It binds to the 50S ribosomal subunit and is static.

CHLORAMPHENICOL produces the "gray baby syndrome" that is often FATAL.

Chloramphenicol is orally absorbed, penetrates the CSF and is inactivated in the liver by conjugation. Infants have a decreased ability to conjugate chloramphenicol, resulting in high levels in the blood. They get abdominal distension, vomiting, cyanosis, hypothermia, decreased respiration, and vasomotor collapse.

CHLORAMPHENICOL is associated with bone marrow depression and aplastic anemia that is usually FATAL.

Chloramphenicol is reserved for life-threatening infections because of serious life-threatening adverse effects. A dose-related bone marrow depression can occur and a dose-related reversible anemia has been reported. An idiosyncratic aplastic anemia can occur that is usually FATAL. Chloramphenicol can also cause hemolytic anemia in G-6-PD–deficient patients.

CLINDAMYCIN

These drugs (clindamycin and lincomycin) are sometimes called *lincosamides* based on their chemical structure. Notice that they end in *-mycin,* but are *not* related to the aminoglycosides or macrolides. Lincomycin is rarely used, so focus on remembering clindamycin.

Clindamycin binds to the 50S ribosomal subunit.

Clindamycin penetrates most tissues, including bone. It has activity against anaerobes and has been associated with pseudomembranous colitis.

Clindamycin has been listed as the drug of choice for anaerobic GI infections. Use of clindamycin is associated with pseudomembranous colitis, since *C. difficile* is resistant to clindamycin.

FOLATE ANTAGONISTS (SULFONAMIDES AND TRIMETHOPRIM)

·

Mechanism of Action

Selected Features

· · · · · · · · · · · · ·

MECHANISM OF ACTION

To understand the mechanism of action of this class of drugs, we need to first review the synthesis of folic acid (Fig. 28-1). Bacteria cannot absorb folic acid, but must make it from PABA (*para*-aminobenzoic acid), pteridine, and glutamate. For humans, folic acid is a vitamin. We cannot synthesize it. This makes this metabolic pathway a nice selective target for antimicrobial agents.

The sulfonamides are structurally similar to PABA and block the incorporation of PABA into dihydropteroic acid. Trimethoprim prevents reduction of dihydrofolate to tetrahydrofolate by inhibiting the dihydrofolate reductase enzyme. This enzyme is present in humans, but trimethoprim has a lower affinity for the human enzyme. There are other examples of folate reductase inhibitors that we will consider later (pyrimethamine and metho-

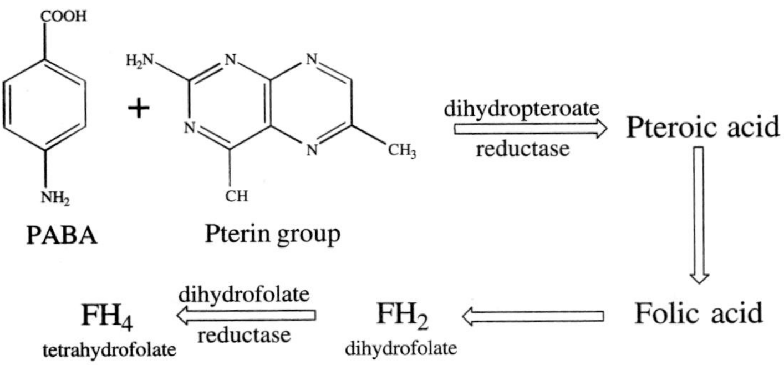

Figure 28-1
This figure presents the synthesis of folic acid, for review.

trexate). The combination of sulfonamides and trimethoprim is synergistic and they are rarely used alone. Sulfamethoxazole is the sulfonamide used in combination with trimethoprim because they have matching half-lives.

SELECTED FEATURES

sulfadiazine	sulfasalazine	TRIMETHOPRIM
sulfisoxazole	SULFAMETHOXAZOLE	co-trimoxazole
sulfapyridine	sulfacetamide	

There are other sulfonamides; please check in your textbook. Note that sulfasalazine is also used to treat inflammatory bowel disease (Chap. 42).

These folate antagonists are broad spectrum agents that are effective against gram-positive and gram-negative organisms.

The combination of sulfamethoxazole and trimethoprim, called co-trimoxazole, is probably the most commonly used drug in this group. It is used for urinary tract infections, *Pneumocystis carinii* pneumonitis, and acute otitis, among other things.

QUINOLONES AND URINARY TRACT ANTISEPTICS

·

Drugs in This Group

Quinolones

Nitrofurantoin

Methenamine

· · · · · · · · · · · ·

DRUGS IN THIS GROUP

The quinolones are a relatively new group of antimicrobials that were originally used primarily to treat urinary tract infections. Therefore, many books often put this grouping together.

Quinolones	
nalidixic acid	norfloxacin
CIPROFLOXACIN	ofloxacin
lomefloxacin	enoxacin
Miscellaneous drugs	
nitrofurantoin	methenamine

QUINOLONES

The quinolones are a relatively new class of drugs, especially the -*floxacins*. For now, the names are easy to recognize, except for nalidixic acid. Hopefully the new ones that appear in the next few years will also be easy to recognize.

The quinolones inhibit DNA synthesis through a specific action on DNA gyrase.

These drugs are considered in a separate category because they have a different structure and a different mechanism of action. They inhibit DNA gyrase and, thus, DNA synthesis. DNA gyrase is the bacterial enzyme that is responsible for the unwinding and supercoiling of DNA. This is the only class of antibacterials that inhibit DNA replication. This is a more common approach for the antivirals and the anticancer drugs.

The most common use for these drugs is in the treatment of urinary tract infections.

These drugs are considered to be broad spectrum antimicrobial agents. Nalidixic acid was the first available and it is an effective urinary tract antiseptic (it sterilizes the urine). The newer agents in this group are useful in a wide range of bacterial infections, including lower respiratory tract infections, bone and joint infections, and prostatitis.

The newer members of this group (ofloxacin and ciprofloxacin) are effective against *Pseudomonas aeruginosa* and are orally active.

CIPROFLOXACIN has found use in the treatment of traveler's diarrhea.

Since these are relatively new drugs, the indications for their use may change over the years, and new agents will probably appear on the market.

NITROFURANTOIN

The mechanism of action of this drug is not clear. It is a broad spectrum antimicrobial that is active after oral administration.

> Nitrofurantoin is used to treat urinary tract infections.

METHENAMINE

> Methenamine is metabolized to formaldehyde and ammonia and is used to treat urinary tract infections.

If you are simply overloaded at this point, skip this drug.

This drug is an interesting example of a prodrug. The parent compound is not active. In acidic pH it is hydrolyzed to ammonia and formaldehyde. The formaldehyde is lethal to bacteria. Therefore, this is another -*cidal* drug. Methenamine is usually administered as a salt of an acid to help keep the pH of the urine less than 5.5, which is vital for the effective use of methenamine.

DRUGS USED TO TREAT TUBERCULOSIS AND LEPROSY

·

Class Organization

Isoniazid

Rifampin

Ethambutol

Pyrazinamide

Dapsone and the Treatment of Leprosy

· · · · · · · · · · · ·

CLASS ORGANIZATION

The mycobacteria that cause tuberculosis and leprosy are very slow growing, so therapy must be continued for relatively long periods of time. To prevent the emergence of resistant strains it is vital to employ combined therapy with at least two agents to which the organism is sensitive.

The drugs are most commonly divided into two groups: first-line drugs and second-line drugs. For most purposes, knowledge of the first-line drugs is adequate. If you decide to specialize in infectious disease or the treatment of tuberculosis, then a working knowledge of the other drugs is important.

FIRST-LINE DRUGS	SECOND-LINE DRUGS
ISONIAZID	aminosalicylic acid
RIFAMPIN	capreomycin
ETHAMBUTOL	cycloserine
pyrazinamide	ethionamide
streptomycin	kanamycin

Some textbooks do not include streptomycin with the first-line drugs. It was covered in more detail in Chap. 27, so we will not consider it again. Take one second to notice that several of the second-line drugs are *-mycins*. Now concentrate your time on the first-line drugs.

ISONIAZID

ISONIAZID inhibits synthesis of mycolic acids.

Isoniazid has a very simple structure. It works on mycobacteria by inhibiting the synthesis of mycolic acids that are unique to the mycobacteria. The mycolic acids are constituents of the bacterial cell envelope.

There are fast and slow acetylators of ISONIAZID.

You may have already heard mention of fast and slow acetylators. This is a genetically determined trait. Acetylation is a metabolic pathway for many drugs, but this pathway is of particular importance for isoniazid. Isoniazid has a shorter half-life in fast acetylators.

ISONIAZID is associated with hepatotoxicity and peripheral neuropathy.

Hepatitis is the most severe side effect of isoniazid. Isoniazid-induced liver dysfunction (as measured by liver function tests) can occur in 10 to 20 percent of patients and the incidence increases with age. The liver dysfunction is reversible in most patients.

The peripheral neuropathy results from pyridoxine deficiency. This results from a chemical combination of isoniazid and pyridoxine. The deficiency can be corrected by pyridoxine supplementation.

ISONIAZID is the DRUG OF CHOICE for chemoprophylaxis in recent convertors.

If a person has had negative TB tests (PPD test, purified protein derivative) in the past, and then one year the test is positive, that person is said to be a recent convertor. The current recommendations (of course, subject to change) is that the person be placed on isoniazid, as long as there is no evidence of clinical disease, such as a positive chest radiography.

RIFAMPIN

RIFAMPIN inhibits RNA synthesis by formation of a stable complex with DNA-dependent RNA polymerase.

Rifampin binds to the β subunit of DNA-dependent RNA polymerase. The complex that is formed is inactive, thus blocking RNA synthesis. Resistance to rifampin is due to a single-step mutation that results in an alteration of the β subunit.

RIFAMPIN is metabolized in the liver and is a potent inducer of the P-450 enzymes. It can cause hepatitis and will color secretions red-orange.

Rifampin is deacetylated in the liver to an active metabolite. A drug-induced hepatitis can occur that results in jaundice. In addition, rifampin will induce the liver microsomal P-450 enzymes. This can lead to increased metabolism of any other drug that is also metabolized by this system.

Rifampin may color urine, feces, saliva, sweat, and tears red-orange. The color can even get into contact lenses.

ETHAMBUTOL

ETHAMBUTOL can cause optic neuritis.

The mechanism of action of ethambutol is unknown. However, it has an interesting adverse effect that often appears on exams. Ethambutol can cause optic neuritis, resulting in loss of central vision and impaired red-green discrimination. It is often suggested that patients have a thorough eye exam before beginning treatment. Ethambutol may also increase serum levels of uric acid due to decreased renal clearance of urate. The increased serum levels of uric acid may lead to gout.

PYRAZINAMIDE

Pyrazinamide is effective against intracellular organisms. It increases levels of serum uric acid.

Pyrazinamide has some features in common with ethambutol. You can make associations, but do not confuse the drugs. The mechanism of action of pyrazinamide is unknown. Pyrazinamide is particularly effective against intracellular organisms. Hyperuricemia occurs in all patients and may result in gout. Pyrazinamide has also been associated with hepatotoxicity.

DAPSONE AND THE TREATMENT OF LEPROSY

The treatment of leprosy is a very specialized area.

The only medical use of DAPSONE has been for the treatment of leprosy.

For years dapsone was the mainstay of the treatment of leprosy. However, the problem of drug-resistance worldwide is becoming severe. Therefore current recommendations (of course, subject to change) is that all forms of leprosy be treated with a combination of drugs.

Dapsone is a structural analog of PABA and is a competitive inhibitor of folic acid synthesis.

Rifampin is an active antileprosy drug as well as anti-TB drug.

ANTIFUNGAL DRUGS
·

Class Organization

Polyene Antifungals

Azole Antifungals

Flucytosine

Griseofulvin

Nystatin

CLASS ORGANIZATION

Many fungal infections occur in poorly vascularized tissues or avascular structures such as the superficial layer of the skin, nails and hair. Fungi are slow growing and are therefore more difficult to kill than bacteria where cell division can be a target for the antimicrobials. Host factors play an important role in determining prognosis with fungal infections, since many fungi are opportunistic. The antifungal agents essentially assist the host immune system with the fight against the fungus.

In general these drugs are poorly soluble, and therefore distribution to the site of action is often a problem. Consider these issues as you study these drugs. As with the antimicrobials consider the host versus invading organism issue. The drug should only attack the invading/foreign organism and not attack the host/human cells.

Classification can be done in a couple of ways. One of the most obvious ways to classify these drugs is by whether they are active against systemic fungal infections or superficial fungal infections. The systemic infections include diseases like disseminated blastomycosis or coccidioidomycosis. The superficial mycoses include infections with dermatophytes of the skin, hair, and nails.

SYSTEMIC FUNGAL INFECTIONS	SUPERFICIAL INFECTIONS
AMPHOTERICIN B	griseofulvin
flucytosine	nystatin
ketoconazole	clotrimazole
miconazole	econazole
fluconazole	butoconazole
itraconazole	oxiconazole
	terconazole
	naftifine
	tolnaftate

Notice that many of the drugs in the list above end in -azole. They are all chemically related and have many features in common. Thus, a better classification may be to relate all of the compounds and then consider the others.

AZOLES	POLYENES	OTHERS
imidazoles (2N)	amphotericin B	flucytosine
topical	nystatin	griseofulvin
clotrimazole		naftifine
econazole		tolnaftate
butoconazole		
sulconazole		
oxiconazole		
topical and systemic		
ketoconazole		
miconazole		
triazoles (3N)		
systemic		
itraconazole		
terconazole		
fluconazole		

This organizes the antifungals by mechanism of action. This is probably an easier way to categorize these drugs in your mind. This way when new drugs are developed you have a place to file the information in your brain.

POLYENE ANTIFUNGALS

> The polyene antifungals, AMPHOTERICIN B and nystatin, work by binding to ergosterol, the principal fungal membrane sterol.

Amphotericin B is the most common antifungal agent and the one that you should know better than the rest. However, remember that nystatin is also a polyene compound and has the same mechanism of action. Both drugs work by an interaction with ergosterol, the principal fungal membrane sterol. Mammalian cells also contain sterols (principally cholesterol). However, ergosterol has a greater affinity for amphotericin than does cholesterol. Once the drug has bound to the ergosterol, there is a disruption of membrane function and electrolytes can leak from the cell.

Although it is not important to memorize the structures of any of these compounds, do take a moment and look at the structure of amphotericin B in your textbook.

> The most serious and most common toxicity of AMPHOTERICIN B is nephrotoxicity.

The nephrotoxicity is related to dose and duration of therapy.

> AMPHOTERICIN B is not absorbed from the GI tract, so it must be given intravenously or topically.

AZOLE ANTIFUNGALS

The azoles are so named because of the azole ring structure that is part of each of these drugs (Fig. 31-1). They are divided into two groups: the

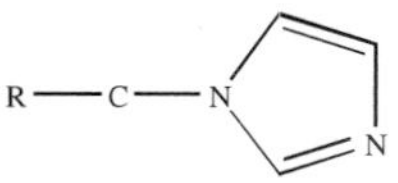

azole ring with
2 nitrogens

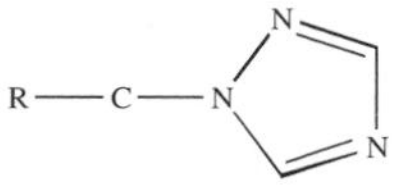

azole ring with
3 nitrogens

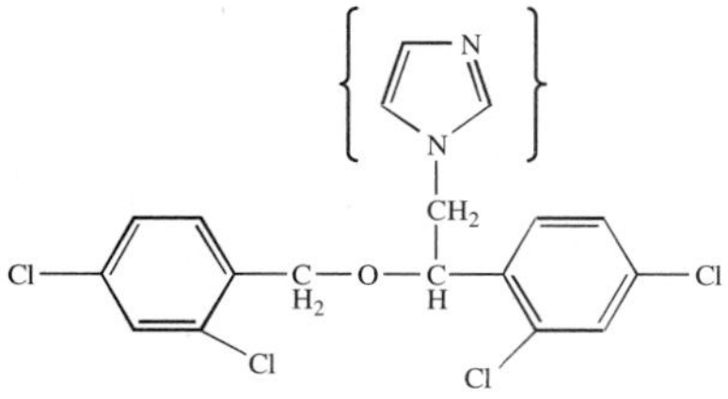

miconazole

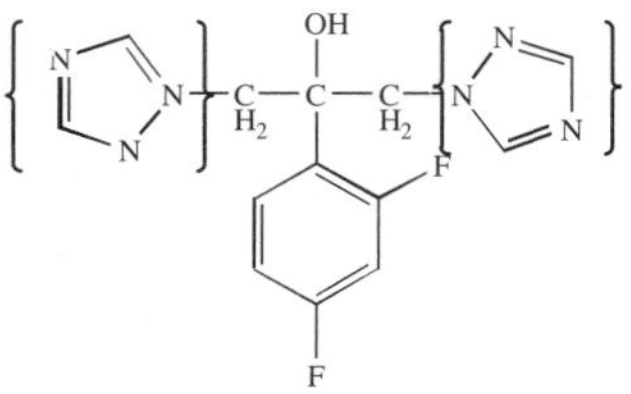

fluconazole

Figure 31-1
On the left is shown the imidazoles with two nitrogens in the azole ring, and on the right is shown the triazoles with three nitrogens in the azole ring.

imidazoles with two nitrogens in the azole ring, and the triazoles with three nitrogens in the ring. Notice that the names *all* end in *-azole*. This makes recognition of these agents simple.

The azole antifungal agents work by inhibiting synthesis of ergosterol.

The exact mechanism is probably not that important, but be sure to read it quickly in your book—the general idea is that these drugs mess with the fungal ergosterol.

Name recognition and mechanism of action are the most important points for these drugs. If you have time and energy, add some facts about the individual agents.

FLUCYTOSINE

Of the other antifungal agents, two are particularly important and should be familiar to you. They are flucytosine and griseofulvin.

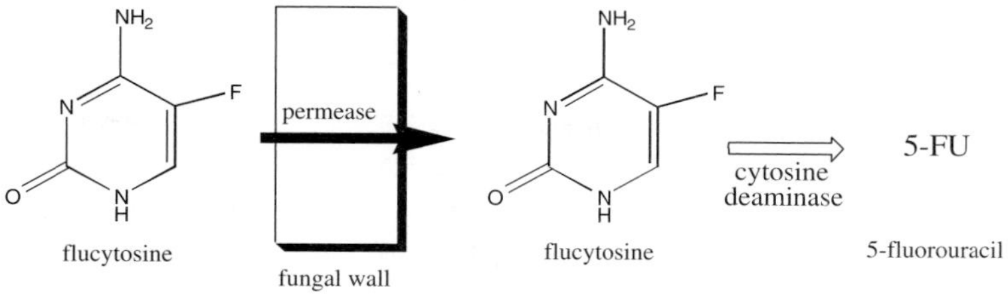

Figure 31-2
Remember that flucytosine enters the cell via a transport protein and then is metabolized to the active compound.

Flucytosine (5-fluorocytosine) is a fluorinated pyrimidine that acts as an antimetabolite.

The mechanism of action of flucytosine should be reminiscent of other antimetabolites. The only special consideration is that it is an antimetabolite for fungus.

Flucytosine enters the cell via a transport protein called *cytosine permease* (Fig. 31-2). Inside the cell it is deaminated by an enzyme (cytosine deaminase) to an active metabolite, 5-fluorouracil. If you have had anticancer drugs this should look very familiar to you. 5-Fluorouracil is further metabolized to an active metabolite that inhibits thymidylate synthetase and inhibits DNA synthesis. The key here is that mammalian cells do not have the cytosine deaminase enzyme.

Additional facts about flucytosine may be important. For example, flucytosine is well absorbed after oral administration and is widely distributed. It readily penetrates the CNS. It is not metabolized and is excreted by glomerular filtration in the kidney.

GRISEOFULVIN

Griseofulvin is administered orally for treatment of superficial fungal infections.

This is a very interesting drug from the point of view of drug administration. The target tissues are those that are not well vascularized: hair, skin, and nails. Yet this drug is given orally and not applied topically.

Griseofulvin specifically binds to keratin in keratin precursor cells making them resistant to fungal infections. A dermatophyte infection can only be cured when infected skin, nails, or hair is replaced by the new keratin-containing griseofulvin. This is why treatment must be continued for long periods of time.

Griseofulvin binds to microtubules and alters the processing of new cell wall needed for fungal growth.

The drug enters susceptible fungi through an energy-dependent transport system and inhibits mitosis.

If you are doing great and want to add one more fact, try this one.

NYSTATIN

Nystatin use is restricted to the topical treatment of candidiasis.

ANTHELMINTICS

·

Class Organization

Treatment of Cestodes and Trematodes

Treatment of Nematodes

Treatment of Filaria

· · · · · · · · · · · ·

CLASS ORGANIZATION

These drugs are effective against worms (helminths). In humans the worms may remain within the intestinal lumen or may have complex life cycles that involve movement through the body. The infective form may be either an adult worm or an immature worm.

The worm life cycle is strongly dependent on neuromuscular coordination, energy production, and microtubular integrity. Most antiworm drugs target one of these three areas.

The easiest way to organize these drugs is to consider a reasonable organization of the worms. The helminths (worms) are classified into three groups: the cestodes (flatworms), nematodes (roundworms), and the trematodes (flukes). If you look at a table of worms and the drug of choice for each worm, several patterns emerge.

TREATMENT OF CESTODES AND TREMATODES

Trematodes (flukes) are treated (for the most part) by PRAZI-QUANTEL.

Cestodes (tapeworms) are treated (for the most part) by NICLOSAMIDE and PRAZIQUANTEL.

Let's stop and consider these two drugs before moving on to the more complex nematodes. First, a quick review of the worms. Cestodes are the tapeworms. They are flat and segmented. The head has suckers. The larvae develop into adults in the small intestine. Therefore, treatment can stay in the small intestine.

The trematodes are the flukes. If you recall, the flukes move about the body—there are blood flukes, liver flukes, and so on. Therefore, the treatment needs to reach the systemic circulation and, thus, the fluke.

NICLOSAMIDE inhibits production of energy and is not absorbed from the GI tract.

Niclosamide inhibits uptake of glucose, which results in a loss of glycogen and decreased ATP synthesis. This does not affect the host since the drug is not absorbed from the GI tract. It is used for cestodes (tapeworms) since a major part of their life cycle involves maturation in the small intestine.

PRAZIQUANTEL paralyzes the worm muscle.

Praziquantel alters the membrane function of the worm and increases membrane permeability. It is absorbed after oral administration. That's why it can have an action on the trematodes (flukes) that cause schistosomiasis.

TREATMENT OF NEMATODES

Nematodes (roundworms) are treated (for the most part) by mebendazole or thiabendazole. The exception is filaria.

The nematodes are a more diverse set of worms. Overall, they are known as the roundworms because they are elongated and cylindrical (round). This group includes whipworm, pinworm and hookworm. Most of them can be treated by thiabendazole or mebendazole (these drugs are related—that's why their names look alike). A special group of nematodes can be considered separately—the filaria. The filaria are treated by two other drugs.

MEBENDAZOLE inhibits protein function in the worms.

Mebendazole binds to tubulin and inhibits glucose uptake. It can be given orally and very little is absorbed from the GI tract.

Thiabendazole inhibits energy production.

Thiabendazole inhibits fumarate reductase (enzyme) and inhibits ATP synthesis. In helminths, but not mammals (including us humans), fumarate is the terminal electron acceptor in anaerobic metabolism. Do you remember the pathway for anaerobic metabolism in humans?

Thiabendazole is absorbed after oral administration.

TREATMENT OF FILARIA

Filariasis is treated (for the most part) with diethylcarbamazine or ivermectin.

Filaria are threadlike worms that are found in blood and tissue. They are transmitted by the bite of a fly or mosquito. Early on they move through the lymphatic system.

DIETHYLCARBAMAZINE enhances phagocytosis of the filaria.

Diethylcarbamazine appears to alter the surface of the filaria in such a way that they are more susceptible to phagocytosis by the host immune system.

Ivermectin paralyzes the worm muscle and is the DRUG OF CHOICE for onchocerciasis (cutaneous filariasis).

Ivermectin is more commonly known in veterinary medicine, but has found a niche in the treatment of onchocerciasis. It appears to block GABA-mediated transmission in the invading organism without any effect on the host.

· C H A P T E R · 3 3 ·

ANTIVIRAL AGENTS

·

Class Organization

Special Features About Some of the Drugs

CLASS ORGANIZATION

There are three basic approaches that are taken to control viral diseases. Vaccination is used to try to prevent and control spread of disease. Chemotherapy (the focus of pharmacology) is used to treat the symptoms of viral illness and to try to eliminate the virus from the body. Finally, stimulation of the host natural resistance mechanisms is used to shorten the duration of illness.

The problems with chemotherapy are similar to those discussed for antimicrobial and antifungal agents. Anytime we are trying to kill an invading/foreign organism there is the problem of the drug recognizing and distinguishing the invading organism from the host.

To understand the antiviral agents, it is necessary to review the life cycle of viruses and imagine sites where drugs could interfere or block this process.

1. Attachment and penetration of the virus to the host cell
2. Uncoating of the viral genome within the host cell

3. Synthesis of viral components within the host cell
4. Assembly of viral particles
5. Release of the virus to spread and invade other cells

Most of the drugs that are currently available block specific viral proteins that are involved in synthesis of viral components within the host cell

Some of the more common antiviral agents are included in the following list. Compare this to your textbook or class notes to be sure which drug names you are responsible for.

EFFECTIVE AGAINST HIV	OTHER ANTIVIRALS
ZIDOVUDINE (AZT) didanosine (DDI) zalcitabine (DDC)	AMANTADINE rimantadine RIBAVIRIN vidarabine (ara-A) acyclovir idoxuridine ganciclovir famciclovir

Notice two things about this list of drugs. First, most of the names end in *-ine* (*-udine, -osine, -adine, -abine*). While this is a very common ending, it should help somewhat in the recognition of these names as belonging to the antiviral group. Second, the list has been divided into drugs effective against HIV and others. This is done because, for now, the target for the HIV drugs is the same.

HIV is the virus that causes AIDS. Hopefully, the list of drugs with some effect against HIV will be longer by the time this book is published. As a reminder, HIV is an RNA retrovirus, which means that it has a specific enzyme called reverse transcriptase. This enzyme is the target of the currently available drugs.

SPECIAL FEATURES ABOUT SOME OF THE DRUGS

ZIDOVUDINE (AZT), didanosine (DDI) and zalcitabine (DDC) all inhibit the formation of viral DNA from RNA by reverse transcriptase.

Zidovudine is a derivative of thymidine that is incorporated into viral DNA during the reverse transcription of the viral RNA. This results in the early termination of DNA elongation. Didanosine is *did*eoxy*i*nosine and is often referred to as DDI. In the cell it is converted to dideoxyadenosine and then dideoxy-ATP. This ATP derivative inhibits the reverse transcriptase. Zalcitabine is *did*eoxy*c*ytidine and is often referred to as DDC. It undergoes a similar transformation to a triphosphate compound, which inhibits the reverse transcriptase.

ACYCLOVIR is used to treat herpes infections. To be effective it must be converted to a phosphorylated derivative.

Acyclovir is used topically, intravenously, and orally for the treatment of herpes infections. Like the HIV antivirals DDI and DDC, acyclovir must undergo a triple phosphorylation to an active derivative. Acyclovir triphosphate inhibits the herpes virus DNA polymerase.

AMANTADINE and rimantadine impair the ability of a virus to uncoat its RNA in host cells.

AMANTADINE is used for the prevention and treatment of influenza type A infections.

RIBAVIRIN is used in the treatment of respiratory syncytial virus (RSV) in infants in young children.

The mechanism of action of ribavirin is unknown, but it is felt to be an antimetabolite. It is used in an aerosol for the treatment of RSV in young children. This could be labeled as a DRUG OF CHOICE.

· C H A P T E R · 3 4 ·

Antiprotozoal Drugs
·

Class Organization

Special Features about Some of the Drugs

Antimalarial Agents

Therapeutic Considerations

Special Features of Some Antimalarials

· · · · · · · · · · · ·

CLASS ORGANIZATION

For simplification we will talk about the antimalarial drugs in a separate section.

Some of the more common protozoal diseases are:

PROTOZOA	DISEASE
Entamoeba histolytica	Amoebiasis: diarrhea
Balantidium coli	Balantidial dysentery
Trichomonas vaginalis	Trichomoniasis: genital infection
Giardia lamblia	Giardiasis: diarrhea
Leishmania	Leishmaniasis: three types
Trypanosoma brucei	African sleeping sickness
Trypanosoma cruzi	Chagas' disease: South American

Of the list of drugs that are used in these diseases, metronidazole is the *one* that is the most important for you to know. This plus a few more trivial facts will get you a long way. You need to be aware of the other drugs and where to find the information about treatment for these diseases.

METRONIDAZOLE	emetine
iodoquinol	dehydroemetine
pentamidine	suramin
eflornithine	nifurtimox
quinacrine	sodium stibogluconate
melarsoprol	

SPECIAL FEATURES ABOUT SOME OF THE DRUGS

METRONIDAZOLE is the most effective agent available for the treatment of all forms of amoebiasis.

Metronidazole is effective against most anaerobic bacteria and several protozoa. It penetrates protozoal and bacterial cell walls, but cannot enter mammalian cells. The drug must be activated once it has entered the cell. The activating enzyme, nitroreductase, is only found in anaerobic organisms. The reduced metronidazole inhibits DNA replication by causing breaks and inhibiting repair of the DNA.

METRONIDAZOLE is effective in the treatment of vaginal trichomoniasis.

Metronidazole is highly effective in the treatment of trichomoniasis. The most common side effects are nausea, vomiting, and diarrhea. It can turn the urine dark or red-brown and cause a metallic taste in the mouth (not the urine). Metronidazole can cause a disulfiram-like reaction when taken with alcohol. The disulfiram-like effect consists of abdominal cramping, vomiting, flushing, or headache after drinking alcohol.

Quinacrine is the DRUG OF CHOICE for giardiasis, but metronidazole is also commonly used.

> Nifurtimox is useful in the treatment of acute Chagas' disease.

Chagas' disease can be fatal, especially if the disease becomes chronic. Therefore, this little fact may be useful to store away.

> Sodium stibogluconate is the DRUG OF CHOICE for all three forms of leishmaniasis.

Sodium stibogluconate is a compound that contains antimony. This is Sb (atomic number 51) on your periodic table of the elements. This is an interesting compound, but don't worry about remembering much about it.

> Suramin is the DRUG OF CHOICE for African trypanosomiasis.

Again, just a drug of choice and not much else to know at this time.

> Iodoquinol is the DRUG OF CHOICE for the treatment of asymptomatic amoebiasis.

These patients do not have symptoms of their *E. histolytica* infection, but are passing amoebic cysts that are potentially infectious.

ANTIMALARIAL AGENTS

Malaria is caused by single cell protozoa of the genus *Plasmodium.* There are over 50 species of *Plasmodium,* but only four are infectious to humans: *P. malariae, P. ovale, P. vivax* and *P. falciparum. P. vivax* is the most prevalent, but *P. falciparum* is the most serious and lethal form of malaria.

To understand the drugs and the rationale behind treatment it is important to understand the life cycle of the malaria organism (Fig. 34-1).

Notice that only *P. vivax* and *P. ovale* can persist in the liver and, therefore, can relapse.

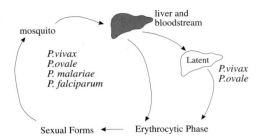

Figure 34-1
As a reminder, the life cycle of the malaria-causing protozoa is presented. The *P. vivax* and *P. ovale* are the two that can take up residence in the liver.

THERAPEUTIC CONSIDERATIONS

It is felt that the symptoms of malaria are due to the erythrocytic form of the parasite. Therefore, elimination of this asexual form will relieve symptoms. Drugs that do this are called *suppressive* or *schizonticidal* agents.

The emergence of chloroquine-resistant organisms is becoming a major health concern. However, the nuances of treatment of resistant organisms will not be addressed here. First, try to understand the whys and wherefores of sensitive organisms. Later in infectious disease learn about the more difficult resistant organisms.

STAGE	EFFECTIVE DRUGS	THERAPEUTIC GOAL
Sporozoites	none	Destroy sporozoites to prevent infection
Primary exoerythrocytic	primaquine	Prevent erythrocytic infection
Secondary exoerythrocytic	primaquine	Prevent relapse
Erythrocytic	quinine chloroquine hydroxychloroquine mefloquine pyrimethamine	Treatment of clinical symptoms
Sexual	primaquine	Prevent spread of infection back to mosquito

Notice on this simplified table that primaquine is used for exoerythrocytic phase (primary and secondary) and to kill gametocytes (sexual phase). All others drugs are erythrocytic. This should make things much easier to remember.

SPECIAL FEATURES OF SOME ANTIMALARIALS

PRIMAQUINE is effective against liver forms (exoerythrocytic) and will kill gametocytes.

Because of its effectiveness against the liver phases, primaquine is often used as prophylaxis. The mechanism of action of primaquine is unknown.

PRIMAQUINE can cause hemolytic anemia in glucose-6-phosphate dehydrogenase deficient patients.

Do you remember the glucose-6-phosphate dehydrogenase enzyme? In biochemistry they probably told you that some people are deficient of this enzyme and should avoid taking certain drugs. Primaquine is one of those drugs. This is an important (albeit somewhat trivial) fact that is important to know.

CHLOROQUINE is the DRUG OF CHOICE for acute uncomplicated attacks of malaria.

Chloroquine is concentrated in the red blood cells, so it is useful to treat the erythrocytic form of malaria. In low doses it is not very toxic. However, in high doses or for long durations of treatment, it can cause toxicity of the skin, blood, and eyes. (NOTE: This is different from the standard nausea, vomiting, and diarrhea). It concentrates in melanin-containing structures and can lead to corneal deposits and blindness.

Quinine is also used for the erythrocytic form of malaria and can be used in chloroquine-resistant disease.

The mechanism of action of quinine is unknown. It is derived from the bark of the cinchona tree, and a name has been given to describe quinine toxicity—cinchonism. Cinchonism consists of sweating, ringing in the ears, impaired hearing, blurred vision, and N, V, D (nausea, vomiting, and diarrhea—for those of you who have not caught on).

Pyrimethamine inhibits dihydrofolate reductase and is used in combination with sulfadoxine.

The plasmodium must synthesize folic acid from PABA, pteridine, and glutamate obtained from the host cell. Pyrimethamine inhibits the conversion of dihydrofolic acid to tetrahydrofolate by preferential binding to the parasite enzyme, dihydrofolate reductase (cf. Fig. 28-1). As with the antibiotics, combination with the sulfonamides provides a sequential blockade of the pathway and a synergistic action. Pyrimethamine is usually combined with sulfadoxine.

ANTICANCER DRUGS

·

Organization of Class

Terminology and General Principles of Therapy

Adverse Effects

Alkylating Agents

Antimetabolites

Antibiotics and Other Natural Products

Hormonal Agents

Miscellaneous Agents

Immunomodulating Agents

Cellular Growth Factors

· · · · · · · · · · · ·

ORGANIZATION OF CLASS

The anticancer drugs usually follow the antimicrobials. This is because the drugs, in many cases, are similar.

Many students get really bogged down with the anticancer drugs. There are an awful lot of drugs with known mechanisms of action and multiple side effects that can be quite serious. However, there are some general principles of the use of these drugs that can be emphasized. In fact, these principles are more important than the individual agents. So for the purposes of this book, focus on name recognition (be sure that you recognize a particular agent as an anti-cancer drug) and a few specific toxicities. Do not try to remember every cancer that the drug is used for on the first pass. You can add some of this information later. Get a handle on the overall picture before you focus on the details.

> Many anticancer drugs have had several names over the years. Don't let this confuse you.

This is another very annoying thing about this group of drugs. Some of these agents are known by several names. I will organize and list drugs in the following table. In parentheses I have tried to include alternate or "old" names. Compare the names and the organization to your textbook or handouts. Highlight or underline the name used in your course.

ALKYLATING AGENTS	ANTIBIOTICS AND OTHER NATURAL PRODUCTS
A. Nitrogen mustards mechlorethamine (nitrogen mustard) cyclophosphamide chlorambucil melphalan ifos famide **B. Nitrosoureas** carmustine lomustine semustine **C. Other alkylating agents** busulfan thiotepa dacarbazine	**A. anthracyclines** doxorubicin daunorubicin (daunomycin) idarubicin **B. other antibiotics** bleomycin mitomycin (mitomycin C) dactinomycin (mithramycin) **C. Vinca alkaloids** vincristine vinblastine **D. other natural products** etoposide teniposide paclitaxel

ANTIMETABOLITES	HORMONAL AGENTS

A. Folate antagonist
  methotrexate
B. Purine analogs
  thioguanine (6-thioguanine)
  mercaptopurine (6-mercaptopurine)
  fludarabine
  pentostatin
  cladribine
C. Pyrimidine analogs
  cytarabine (cytosine arabinoside, ara-C)
  fluorouracil (5-FU)
	A. glucocorticoids
	B. estrogens/antiestrogens
	  tamoxifen citrate
	  estramustine phosphate sodium
	C. androgens/antiandrogens
	  flutamide
	D. LH–RH antagonists
	  leuprolide

MISCELLANEOUS AGENTS	IMMUNOMODULATING AGENTS	CELLULAR GROWTH FACTORS
hydroxyurea procarbazine (N-methyl-hydrazine, ? alkylating) mitotane cisplatin (? alkylating) mitoxantrone asparaginase	interferons	filgrastim (G-CSF) sargramostim (GM-CSF)

There are an awful lot of drugs. Notice that under the antibiotics and natural products there are a number of drugs that end in -*mycin*. Be careful not to confuse these with the "real" antibiotics.

The drugs can be basically divided into two simple groups: the cytotoxic drugs and the hormones. All of the alkylating agents, antibiotics, antimetabolites, and miscellaneous drugs are cytotoxic drugs—they kill cells. Therefore, all of the following terminology and general principles apply to the cytotoxic drugs.

TERMINOLOGY AND GENERAL PRINCIPLES OF THERAPY

Anticancer therapy is aimed at killing dividing cells. There are normal host cells that are also dividing. Effects on these cells cause side effects.

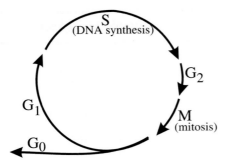

Figure 35-1
Cells go through several cycles
around cell division. DNA synthesis occurs during the S
phase and the actual division
takes place during M phase.

This is a bit simplistic, but will serve our purposes for now. In anti-microbial therapy the object is to kill the invading bacteria without harming the host. In anticancer therapy the object is to kill the cancer cells without harming the normal cells. This is difficult because the cancer cells are also human (or host) cells. The cancer cells are basically human cells that have lost control of cell division. Therefore, anticancer treatment is, in large part, aimed at killing dividing cells. Remember that cells in certain places in the body—the epithelium of the GI tract, hair follicles and bone marrow especially—are dividing continuously. Effects on these dividing cells cause adverse effects.

All of the cytotoxic drugs have a narrow safety margin. This just basically restates the previous paragraph. For these drugs, at doses that are effective against the tumor, the drug also has toxic side effects.

Since many of these drugs target dividing cells the cell cycle is important to remember (Fig. 35-1). Where known, books will list the part of the cell cycle in which a drug has an effect. This is not absolutely critical information for the first pass through the material. However, as you learn more about the tumors and their growth rates, this information should be added.

> The *log kill* is an important concept to understand. The anti-cancer drugs kill a constant fraction of cells instead of an absolute number.

The anticancer drugs act by first-order kinetics (Fig. 35-2). Remember any kinetics? This means that a constant fraction of the cells (say 50 per-cent) are killed by one dose. This is quite different than a constant number of cells being killed. If one dose of the drug kills 50 percent of the tumor cells, then a second dose of the drug will kill 50 percent of the remaining tumor cells. This results in a 75 percent reduction in the number of tumor

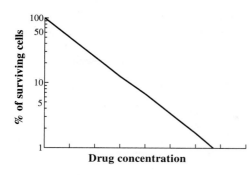

Figure 35-2
There is a linear relationship between the concentration of the anticancer drug and the number of surviving cells, when the number of cells is plotted on a log scale. This means that the anticancer drugs act by first-order kinetics. A constant fraction of cells is killed by each dose of drug.

cells after two doses of this drug. This sort of thinking should remind you very much of pharmacokinetics. The number of tumor cells are usually expressed in exponentials. This is why the "kill" of a drug is described in log units. The drug that reduces the tumor cell load from 10^8 cells to 10^5 cells is said to have achieved a 3 log kill.

> Drug resistance to anticancer drugs is analogous to resistance to antimicrobials.

Cancer cells already contain a mutation that allows unrestricted growth. They can also mutate in a way that makes them resistant to anticancer drugs.

> Combinations of drugs are frequently used in the treatment of cancer.

Combinations of drugs are frequently used to treat cancer. This reduces the incidence of drug resistance. In addition, the drugs used together often target different phases of the cell cycle. The common drug combinations often have acronyms, such as MOPP, VAMP, or POMP, that stand for the individual drugs in the combination. It is not necessary at this time to learn the drug combinations.

ADVERSE EFFECTS

As mentioned above, the adverse effects of these drugs are due to an effect on proliferating cells in the body. We will consider the toxicity of these drugs separately, because the principles behind the toxicity are more important than remembering which drugs have more, or less, of a particular toxicity.

Bone marrow toxicity is due to destruction of proliferating hematopoietic stem cells. This results in a decrease in all blood elements, including white cells and platelets.

Patients on anticancer drugs are at an increased risk of developing life-threatening infections and bleeding. This is due to the decrease in white blood cells and platelets. There are currently available growth factors that can be used to stimulate cell production in the bone marrow (granulocyte colony stimulating factor, granulocyte-macrophage colony stimulating factor, and erythropoietin).

Bleomycin, asparaginase, and the hormonal agents are notable for their lack of significant bone marrow toxicity.

Bone marrow toxicity is so common with these drugs that it is useful to learn the few drugs that do not have significant marrow toxicity.

Gastrointestinal toxicity takes two forms. The nausea and vomiting associated with cancer chemotherapy is felt to be due to a central effect. These drugs can cause damage to the proliferating mucosa of the GI tract.

Almost all of the cancer chemotherapy drugs will cause nausea and vomiting (of course, some are worse than others). It is felt that the drugs stimulate the chemoreceptor trigger zone in the brain, which leads to vomiting. This can be treated with phenothiazines, such as chlorpromazine (see Chap. 20), that block dopamine receptors in this brain region. A serotonin antagonist, ondansetron, has also proved effective in the prevention of nausea and vomiting.

The more predictable effect of the anticancer drugs is the killing of the proliferating cells in the mucosa of the GI tract. Remember that the epithelium of the GI tract is constantly replicating. These drugs kill dividing cells. Therefore, they will damage the epithelium of the GI tract. This can lead to ulcer formation anywhere in the GI tract (mouth, esophagus, stomach, and so on).

> Most anticancer drugs will damage hair follicles and produce hair loss.

This is especially true with cyclophosphamide, doxorubicin, vincristine, methotrexate, and dactinomycin. (Don't worry too much about these now).

> Many of the anticancer drugs can cause local tissue necrosis.

This is important since many of the anticancer drugs are administered intravenously. If any of the drug gets out of the vein there can be severe tissue necrosis. Remember that these are really nasty drugs.

> Renal tubular damage is the major side effect of cisplatin and high-dose methotrexate. Cyclophosphamide can cause hemorrhagic cystitis.

Renal damage is not that common after use of the anticancer drugs. However, it is a significant side effect of a few drugs. Thus, learn these few. For many of the drugs adequate hydration is recommended, but details like this are to be added later.

> Cardiotoxicity is associated with the use of doxorubicin and dauno-rubicin.

Cardiotoxicity is relatively rare with the anticancer drugs. However, there are two drugs that stand out in this category: the two d-orubicins. This particular adverse effect has a habit of showing up on board exams and other such places.

> Bleomycin can cause pulmonary fibrosis, which can be FATAL.

This is another example of a particular drug/adverse effect pair that has a habit of showing up in the most unusual locations. It's not too hard to memorize.

> Vincristine is "known" for its nervous system toxicity.

Vincristine is the only anticancer drug that has a dose-limiting neurotoxicity. Anytime we can use the word ONLY it should register on a memory chip in your brain.

ALKYLATING AGENTS

> All alkylating agents work by adding an alkyl group to DNA.

The drugs in this group all introduce alkyl groups into nucleophilic sites with covalent bonds. There are many sites of alkylation, but the degree of DNA alkylation correlates with the cytotoxicity of the drugs. These drugs are not cycle specific. They are prone to local tissue necrosis and damage.

> The nitrogen mustards include:
> mechlorethamine (used in Hodgkin's)
> cyclophosphamide (hemorrhagic cystitis)
> chlorambucil (drug of choice for chronic lymphocytic leukemia)

I have added a few facts about each of the nitrogen mustards, but the names and the class are more important. If you can add these additional details great, but don't sweat it.

> The nitrosoureas include carmustine, lomustine, and semustine. They are useful in treating brain tumors, because they are lipid-soluble enough to cross the blood–brain barrier.

The nitrosoureas are easy to recognize because of the *-mustine* ending on their names. They are lipid soluble and therefore cross into the central nervous system. They have found use in the treatment of brain tumors. Some books include streptozocin as a nitrosourea. It is different enough (water soluble, renal tubular damage, and islet cell carcinoma of the pancreas) that it is not useful for us to include it here.

The other alkylating agents, busulfan, thiotepa, and dacarbazine should be learned for name recognition only at this time.

ANTIMETABOLITES

The drugs of this group are quite similar to antibiotics and antiviral agents, so they should not be too difficult. They compete for binding sites on enzymes or can be incorporated into DNA or RNA. They are especially useful if they bind to an enzyme that has a major effect on pathways leading to cell replication. That should make sense.

> Methotrexate competitively inhibits dihydrofolate reductase.

Remember this pathway from the antibiotics (cf. Fig. 28-1). Well, methotrexate inhibits the binding of folic acid to the enzyme. It therefore inhibits DNA synthesis by inhibiting thymidylate synthesis. Cellular uptake of methotrexate is by a carrier-mediated active transport. Cellular resistance to methotrexate is presumably due to decreased transport into the cell. This can be overcome by using high doses.

> Leucovorin provides reduced folate to "rescue" normal cells from the action of methotrexate.

Even before you took pharmacology, you had probably heard of leucovorin rescue during cancer treatment. Leucovorin provides cells with reduced folate, thus bypassing the blocked enzyme.

Methotrexate is used to treat psoriasis and severe rheumatoid arthritis in addition to cancer. It can be administered intrathecally. Its major route of elimination is renal.

Just some additional facts about antimetabolites for the brave at heart.

The purine antagonists all have to be activated. They include:
  thioguanine
  mercaptopurine

Compare this activation to the antivirals (Chap. 33).

The pyrimidine antagonists also must be activated. They include:
  cytarabine
  5-fluorouracil

ANTIBIOTICS AND OTHER NATURAL PRODUCTS

The antibiotics all disrupt DNA function.

Most of these drugs bind in some way to DNA.
It is easiest to divide the antibiotics into two groups: the anthracyclines and the others.

The anthracyclines have cardiac toxicity. They include doxorubicin (wide range of tumors) and daunorubicin (acute leukemias)

The anthracyclines are so named because of structure. However, the structure is not of primary importance to us. The cardiac toxicity is the most important thing to know about the *d*-rubicins. Highlight it, make a flash card, do whatever it takes to get you to remember this. The cardiac problems include arrhythmias, decreased function, myofibrillar degeneration, and focal necrosis of myocytes. It is felt that clinical cardiac damage occurs with each dose. It has been postulated that the damage is due to free-radical generation and lipid peroxidation.

Now on to the "other" antibiotics—the *-mycins.*

Bleomycin can cause FATAL pulmonary fibrosis. It does not have significant myelosuppressive effects.

Plicamycin (mithramycin) can be used to treat life-threatening hypercalcemia associated with malignancy.

In addition to its DNA-binding action, plicamycin inhibits resorption of bone by osteoblasts, thus lowering serum calcium. This fact also appears in the oddest of places.

Let us move on to the other plant products, or naturally occurring agents.

The vinca alkaloids (vincristine and vinblastine) bind to tubulin and disrupt the spindle apparatus during cell division.

These two drugs are the most important ones for you to know.

For vincristine, the neurologic toxicity is dose limiting.
For vinblastine, the bone marrow toxicity is dose limiting.

If you can remember that one has neurologic toxicity and one has bone marrow toxicity, then notice that vin*b*lastine is *b*one marrow toxic.

> Paclitaxel is a newer agent that is among the most active of all anti-cancer drugs. It works by preventing depolymerization of micro-tubules.

This drug is relatively new, but you will hear more about it in the years to come. If your textbook is more than several years old, it may not be included.

> Etoposide and teniposide are plant products that do *not* act by binding to microtubules.

These two drugs are further down on the trivia list. Learn the names if you have energy. They are noted here so that you do not generalize the tubulin thing to all the natural plant products.

HORMONAL AGENTS

These drugs are used to treat hormonally sensitive tumors, such as tumors of the breast, prostate, and uterus. The side effects of the drugs are related to the hormonal changes that they induce and not to cytotoxic actions. Obviously, the tumor must have receptors for the hormones in order for the drugs to have an action.

> Tamoxifen is a competitive antagonist of the estrogen receptor. It is used in the treatment of breast cancer.

> Flutamide is a competitive testosterone antagonist that is used to treat prostate cancer.

The LH–RH antagonists (the most common one is leuprolide) block gonadotropin release and this results in decreased estrogen and testosterone production.

Luteinizing hormone–releasing hormone controls the release of gonadotropins. Blocking LH–RH will result in a decrease in estrogen and testosterone. This is similar to the effect of the estrogen or testosterone antagonists. The LH–RH antagonists are used in the treatment of prostate cancer. Initial treatment with leuprolide can cause a transient increase in testosterone production, so it is often used in combination with flutamide.

MISCELLANEOUS AGENTS

There are numerous other anticancer drugs. Some of these are occasionally classified as alkylating agents (procarbazine and cisplatin). Please compare to your textbook or class handouts.

Cisplatin has a dose-limiting renal toxicity.

Cisplatin is the miscellaneous drug that is listed most often in pharmacology textbooks. Learn it first. It you can handle more, learn the names of some of the other miscellaneous drugs.

Hydroxyurea inhibits ribonucleotide reductase.
Mitotane is used to treat adrenocortical adenocarcinoma.
Carboplatin is an analog of cisplatin.

IMMUNOMODULATING AGENTS

Modulating the immune system to help in getting rid of tumor cells is an active area of research. The goal is to enhance T-cell function and natural killer cells. Thus, new drugs in the future will probably appear in this class. For now, some name recognition is probably all that is needed.

If you want to start on the trivial facts, interferons are used in the treatment of hairy cell leukemia.

CELLULAR GROWTH FACTORS

This is also an area of research. Hopefully new drugs will also appear in this group. The idea is to stimulate the stem cells in the bone marrow to accelerate recovery from the cytotoxic drugs. Therefore, these drugs are sort-of adjunct to the anticancer drugs that we have been discussing.

If you want to start on the trivial facts, fil*gra*s*tim* (*g*ranulocyte colony *stim*ulating factor) is used to accelerate recovery of neutrophils and sar*gra*mo*stim* (*g*ranulocyte-*m*acrophage colony *stim*ulating factor) is used to accelerate bone marrow repopulation after chemotherapy, radiation, and bone marrow transplantation.

DRUGS THAT AFFECT
THE ENDOCRINE SYSTEM

·

ADRENOCORTICAL HORMONES

·

Organization of Class

Glucocorticoids

Mineralocorticoids

Inhibitors of Adrenocorticoid Synthesis

·　·　·　·　·　·　·　·　·　·　·　·

ORGANIZATION OF CLASS

The term *steroid* relates to the main structural frame of this series of compounds (Fig. 36-1).

The steroid compounds produced by the adrenal cortex are called *adrenal corticosteroids* and they can be divided into two main groups depending on their relative metabolic (glucocorticoid) versus electrolyte-regulating (mineralocorticoid) activity. Of course, each compound will have effects on both metabolism and electrolyte balance, but one effect is usually more potent than the other. Almost every cell in the body will respond to these compounds.

237

GLUCOCORTICOIDS	EQUAL POTENCY	MINERALO-CORTICOIDS
PREDNISONE prednisolone methylprednisolone triamcinolone betamethasone DEXAMETHASONE paramethasone	CORTISOL HYDROCORTISONE	fludrocortisone

Compare this list of drugs with the list in your textbook or class hand-outs. Make any necessary changes to the list.

HYDROCORTISONE (cortisol) is the main glucocorticoid produced by the adrenal.

Notice that hydrocortisone and its close relative, cortisol, are the ONLY two drugs that have equal metabolic (glucocorticoid) and electro-

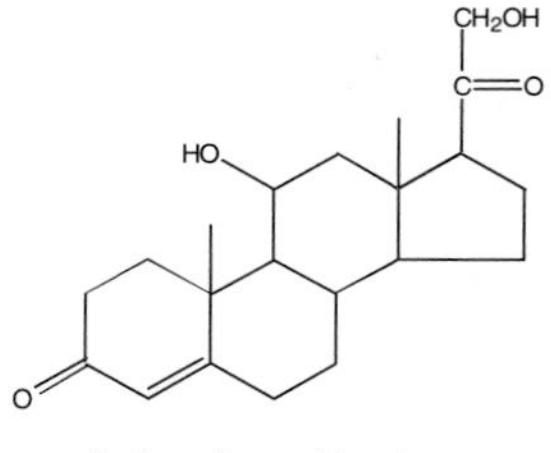

Basic corticosteroid nucleus

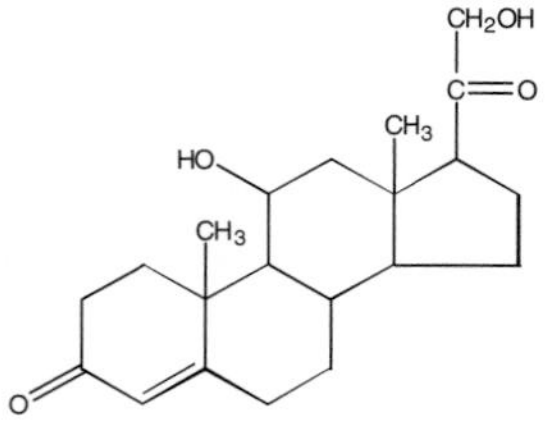

corticosterone 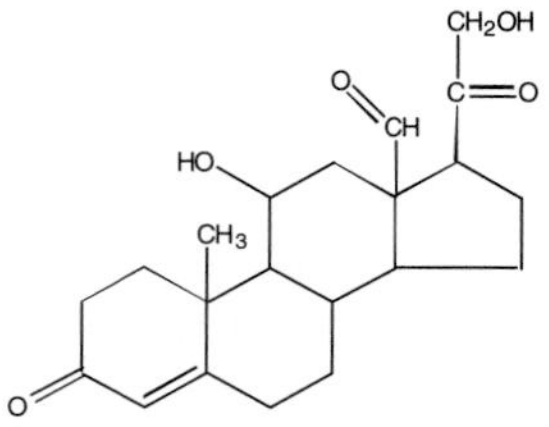   aldosterone

Figure 36-1
The main steroid structure is shown, along with two examples of adrenocortical hormones.

lyte balance (mineralocorticoid) actions. Remember this. Next notice that there are many more drugs listed on the left (glucocorticoid) than on the right (mineralocorticoid). Therefore, if you have to guess about a drug, guess glucocorticoid. Better yet, just learn the mineralocorticoid drug on the right (it starts with "f").

Aldosterone is the main mineralocorticoid produced by the adrenal.

It is useful at this point to review some of the anatomy and physiology of the adrenal gland, with a particular emphasis on the adrenal cortex (Fig. 36-2). The zona glomerulosa (outer layer) produces the compounds that control electrolyte balance, such as aldosterone. The zona fasciculata (middle layer) produces the compounds that regulate metabolism, such as hydrocortisone. The zona reticularis (inner layer) produce sex hormones (Chap. 37). The pituitary hormone ACTH controls the secretions from primarily the inner two layers. The production of mineralocorticoids is mainly controlled by the renin-angiotensin system.

The pharmacological actions of steroids are an extension of their physiologic effects.

This should seem self-evident, but sometimes it is forgotten.

All of the steroids (including the sex steroids) bind to intracellular receptors in target tissues.

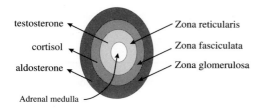

testosterone — Zona reticularis
cortisol — Zona fasciculata
aldosterone — Zona glomerulosa
Adrenal medulla

Figure 36-2
This figure reminds you of the layers of the adrenal cortex and the hormones that each layer produces.

After entering the cell and binding to the receptor, the receptor–hormone complex is transported into the nucleus where it influences RNA synthesis. The actions of the glucocorticoids and mineralocorticoids will be reviewed separately.

GLUCOCORTICOIDS

Glucocorticoids promote normal metabolism.

The glucocorticoids stimulate formation of glucose and inhibit protein synthesis. The net effect is an antagonism of the action of insulin.

Glucocorticoids inhibit inflammatory and immunological responses. This is the basis of their therapeutic use and the reason why patients on glucocorticoids have increased susceptibility to infections.

Glucocorticoids are used for replacement therapy in patients with malfunctioning adrenal glands. But, the most important use of glucocorticoids is to reduce inflammation or block immunological responses. All steps in the inflammatory process are blocked.

Glucocorticoids have a number of other actions. You should read about them, but do not try to memorize them early on. Remember that these compounds will affect nearly every cell in the body.

The complications of glucocorticoid therapy appear in all organ systems.

This should be intuitive. Since the glucocorticoids affect nearly every cell in the body, the adverse effects can arise from nearly every cell in the body. Short-term use (e.g., status asthmaticus) is generally safe. It's long-term use that poses particular problems.

A potentially serious complication of long-term use is osteoporosis.

Glucocorticoids affect bone metabolism in a number of ways. The final result is a decrease in calcification.

Glucocorticoids are reversibly bound to a specific α-globulin called *transcortin,* or *corticosteroid-binding globulin.* The steroids are, for the most part, metabolized in the liver.

MINERALOCORTICOIDS

The mineralocorticoids are involved in salt and water balance.

The mineralocorticoids increase the rate of sodium reabsorption and potassium excretion. The primary site of this action is the distal tubule.

INHIBITORS OF ADRENOCORTICOID SYNTHESIS

Metyrapone and aminoglutethimide will inhibit adrenalcorticoid synthesis.

Name recognition is the most important thing here. If you have time and energy, add the mechanisms of action.

Aminoglutethimide and metyrapone inhibit the conversion of cholesterol to pregnenolone by an enzyme called 11-β-hydroxylase (the rate-limiting step in steroid synthesis). Ketoconazole, an antifungal agent, and spironolactone, an antagonist of aldosterone, will also inhibit adrenal hormone synthesis.

SEX STEROIDS

·

Organization of Class

Estrogens

Antiestrogens

Progestins

Antiprogestins

Oral Contraceptives

Androgens

Antiandrogens

·   ·   ·   ·   ·   ·   ·   ·   ·   ·   ·   ·   ·

ORGANIZATION OF CLASS

Sex hormones are produced by the gonads and the adrenal medulla. The synthesis and release of the hormones are controlled by the anterior pituitary (LH and FSH) and the hypothalamus (gonadotropin-releasing hormone).

> The sex steroids are used therapeutically for replacement therapy and for contraception.

243

These drugs are really very easy to organize.

```
Estrogens
   ESTRADIOL
   estrone
   estriol
   DIETHYLSTILBESTROL
   quinestrol
   ethinyl estradiol
   mestranol
Antiestrogens
   CLOMIPHENE
   TAMOXIFEN
Progestins
   PROGESTERONE
   medroxyprogesterone
   norethindrone
   hydroxyprogesterone
   norgestrol
   megestrol
Antiprogestins
   MIFEPRISTONE
Androgens
   TESTOSTERONE (several preparations)
   methyltestosterone
   fluoxymesterone
   DANAZOL
   testolactone
Antiandrogens
   cyproterone acetate
   flutamide (receptor antagonist)
   FINASTERIDE (5α-reductase inhibitor)
```

First, compare these drug names to those in your textbook or class handouts. The androgens listed here are only the androgenic steroids. I have not included the agents used primarily as anabolic agents. Do not be afraid to cross off drugs on this list if they do not appear in your textbook. Next, look at each name and decide whether you recognize it for what it is (i.e., do you know that norgestrol is a progestin?). All those you are not sure of, put in your list for name recognition. The rest of this is a piece of cake, especially if you remember your endocrine physiology (Fig. 37-1).

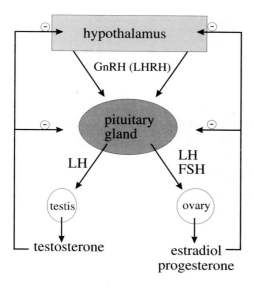

Figure 37-1
This is a very simplified scheme to remind you of the regulation of the sex steroids. There is additional positive and negative feedback to the pituitary. GnRH is gonadotropin-releasing hormone, which is sometimes called LH–RH (leutenizing hormone–releasing hormone).

ESTROGENS

> The major estrogens produced by the body are estradiol, estrone, and estriol.

The ovary is the primary source of estradiol. Estrone and estriol are metabolites of estradiol, courtesy of the liver.

> The most common use of estrogens is in oral contraceptives, but they are also used as replacement therapy in postmenopausal women.

Estrogen therapy combined with progestins are used to block ovulation and prevent pregnancy. In postmenopausal women, estrogens are used to reduce the symptoms of menopause and to reduce osteoporosis. Hormone replacement therapies can slow bone loss, but cannot reverse existing deficits.

> The most common side effects of estrogens are nausea and vomiting.

Estrogens can also cause breast tenderness, endometrial hyperplasia, hyperpigmentation, edema (sodium and water retention) and weight gain. The side effects of estrogens in postmenopausal women tend to be less troublesome because lower doses are used.

> DIETHYLSTILBESTROL (a nonsteroid molecule) has been associated with cervical and vaginal carcinoma in daughters of women that took the drug during pregnancy.

ANTIESTROGENS

There are two important estrogen antagonists, tamoxifen and clomiphene. Neither compound has a steroid structure. Tamoxifen is used in the treatment of breast cancer that has estrogen receptors and is covered in more detail in the anticancer chapter.

> CLOMIPHENE stimulates ovarian function and is used in the treatment of infertility.

Clomiphene interferes with the inhibitory feedback of estrogens on the pituitary and hypothalamus. This results in an increase in the release of gonadotropin-releasing hormone and gonadotropins and stimulation of ovarian function.

PROGESTINS

> PROGESTERONE is the main natural progestin.

Progesterone is produced in the corpus luteum and placenta. Its job is to maintain the uterine endometrium in the secretory phase.

> The major use of progestins is in contraception.

Other clinical uses of progestins include dysfunctional uterine bleeding, suppression of postpartum lactation, treatment of dysmenorrhea, and the management of endometriosis.

> The most common side effects of progestin use are weight gain, edema, and depression.

Increased clotting may also occur, leading to thrombophlebitis or pulmonary embolism.

ANTIPROGESTINS

To date there is only one progestin antagonist—MIFEPRISTONE (RU-486).

ORAL CONTRACEPTIVES

> The most common pharmacological means of preventing pregnancy is the use of estrogens and progestins to interfere with ovulation.

The mechanism of action of the oral contraceptives is not completely understood. The estrogen provides negative feedback on the pituitary inhibiting further release of LH and FSH. This will prevent ovulation. The progestin will also inhibit LH and is added to stimulate withdrawal bleeding.

> Progestin alone in pill form (mini-pill) or implants will also provide contraception.

The use of progestin alone is associated with irregular uterine bleeding.

The side effects of the oral contraceptives are related to the estrogens and progestins that are part of the pills.

Hopefully, you said "Wait, that's obvious!" The major side effects of the combination pills are breast fullness, nausea and vomiting (estrogen) and depression and edema (progestin). There is an increased incidence of abnormal clotting in women who smoke and are over the age of 35.

ANDROGENS

The androgens will have masculinizing and anabolic effects in both men and women. The anabolic effects include: increased muscle mass, increased bone density, and increased red blood cell mass. The virilizing effects include: spermatogenesis, sexual dysfunction, and sexual restoration and development. It is possible to separate (somewhat) the virilizing and anabolic activities by altering the structure of the steroid.

TESTOSTERONE is the major androgen produced in the body.

Testosterone is produced by the Leydig cells of the testes and by the ovaries and adrenal glands. The secretion of testosterone is controlled by hormonal signals from the hypothalamus and anterior pituitary.

The primary therapeutic use of androgens is for replacement therapy in patients with testicular deficiency.

Although the most common use of the androgens is for replacement therapy, other uses do occur. Androgens can be used to stimulate linear bone growth and in the treatment of anemia.

> In women, androgens can be used in the treatment of advanced or metastatic breast cancer. DANAZOL is used in the treatment of endometriosis.

> The side effects of the androgens are related to their physiologic actions.

Simple enough. Androgens will cause virilization of women, including acne, growth of facial hair, deepening of the voice, and excessive muscle development. In men, androgens will block release of gonadotropins and the excess androgens will be converted to estrogens. This may result in azoospermia (too few sperm), impotence and gynecomastia. Excess androgens can also cause liver abnormalities and psychotic episodes. In children, androgens will cause closure of epiphyseal plates and abnormal sexual maturation. These should all make sense and do not need to be memorized.

ANTIANDROGENS

Competitive antagonists of testosterone include cyproterone acetate and flutamide. These drugs have been used to treat excessive hair growth in women and prostate cancer in men.

> FINASTERIDE is a 5α-reductase inhibitor that is used to treat benign prostatic hypertrophy.

5α-reductase converts testosterone to dihydrotestosterone. Dihydrotestosterone is the major intracellular androgen in most target tissues. Finasteride is effective in suppressing accessory function without interfering with libido (mediated by testosterone).

THYROID AND ANTITHYROID DRUGS

·

Organization of Class

Thyroid Replacement Therapy

Drugs That Are Thyroid Downers

· · · · · · · · · · · ·

ORGANIZATION OF CLASS

These drugs are really quite simple if you can recognize the names and if you remember how the thyroid gland is controlled and how it synthesizes thyroid hormone (Fig. 38-1).

The thyroid gland helps maintain an adequate level of metabolism in tissues. Hypothyroidism (low levels of hormone) results in slow heart rate (bradycardia), cold intolerance, and physical slowing. In children, hypothyroidism can result in mental retardation and short stature. Hyperthyroidism (too much hormone) results in fast heart rate, nervousness, tremor, and excess heat production.

> The thyroid gland stores thyroid hormone as thyroglobulin.

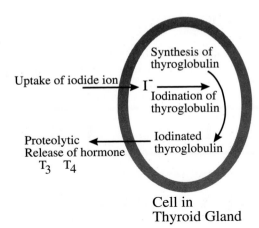

Uptake of iodide ion

Synthesis of thyroglobulin

I⁻

Iodination of thyroglobulin

Proteolytic Release of hormone
T₃ T₄

Iodinated thyroglobulin

Cell in
Thyroid Gland

Figure 38-1
In each thyroid cell there is active uptake of iodide. This iodide is then incorporated onto tyrosine residues in the protein thyroglobulin. The iodinated thyroglobulin then undergoes proteolysis to release thyroid hormone in the form of T_3 and T_4.

THYROID REPLACEMENT THERAPY

There are two major thyroid hormones, called T_3 and T_4. T_3 is the most active form.

T_4 is the major secretory product of the thyroid gland. T_3 is secreted by the thyroid, but is also synthesized by extrathyroid metabolism of T_4. Both T_4 and T_3 are bound to thyroxine-binding globulin and several other proteins in the plasma. T_4 is often referred to as *thyroxine* and T_3 as *triiodothyronine*.

Drugs used in the management of hypothyroidism:
    LEVOTHYROXINE (sodium salt of T_4; most common)
    liothyronine (sodium salt of T_3)
    liotrix (mixture of T_3 and T_4)

LEVOTHYROXINE is the DRUG OF CHOICE for the treatment of hypothyroidism.

DRUGS THAT ARE THYROID DOWNERS

Treatment of hyperthyroidism is achieved by removing part, or all, of the thyroid gland, inhibiting synthesis of thyroid hormone, or by blocking release of hormone from the gland.

Surgery or radioactive iodine can be used to destroy the thyroid gland.

Remember that iodine is taken up selectively by the thyroid gland. Therefore, administration of radioactive iodine will result in the accumulation of radioactivity in the thyroid gland. This is very selective radiation therapy.

PROPYLTHIOURACIL and methimazole will inhibit thyroid synthesis.

Propylthiouracil and methimazole will inhibit iodination of tyrosine groups and coupling of these groups to form thyroid hormone. They have no effect on the stored thyroglobulin or on the release of thyroid hormone. Therefore, there will be a delay between the onset of therapy and the clinical effect as the previously stored thyroglobulin is released.

· C H A P T E R · 3 9 ·

INSULIN, GLUCAGON, AND ORAL HYPOGLYCEMIC DRUGS

·

Organization of Class

Insulins

Oral Hypoglycemic Agents

· · · · · · · · · · · ·

ORGANIZATION OF CLASS

High glucose stimulates an increase in insulin release from β cells of the pancreas. Insulin then drives carbohydrate into cells. Patients that have high glucose levels in their blood are said to have diabetes mellitus.

Of course, you remember that diabetes mellitus is divided into two groups: Type I (insulin dependent) and Type II (non-insulin dependent). These distinctions are important for pharmacology because they make it easier to remember the mechanism of action of the drugs used to treat diabetes mellitus.

As an aside, there is another diabetes that students sometimes confuse with diabetes mellitus, and that is diabetes insipidus. This is a disorder of water and sodium balance. Generally, if someone says "diabetes" they mean the sugar (mellitus) one and not diabetes insipidus.

Back to the topic at hand.

Type I diabetes is related to loss of insulin-secreting cells in the pancreas. Type II diabetes is related to target cell resistance to the action of insulin.

This, of course, is somewhat simplified. An endocrinologist would cringe. The Type I diabetics are dependent on an exogenous (outside the body) source of insulin. This disorder generally appears in childhood, hence the term *juvenile diabetes.* Type II diabetes has been called *adult onset.* It appears to have a genetic basis and the patients are often obese. Type II diabetes is treated with oral agents that will lower blood glucose (hypoglycemics) and with insulin.

That said, we should organize our drugs into insulin and the oral hypoglycemic agents.

INSULINS

Insulin is a small protein of 51 amino acids that is synthesized and secreted by the β cells of the pancreas. Insulin for replacement therapy can be isolated from animal sources. Human insulin is made using recombinant DNA technology.

INSULIN must be administered by injection.

All peptides are degraded by enzymes in the GI tract, so it is not possible to administer insulin by the oral route. Given intravenously it has a half-life of less than 10 minutes (short). Therefore, it is administered subcutaneously.

The most common adverse effect of insulin is hypoglycemia.

I hope that this is intuitively obvious!!

> Insulin preparations vary in their time to onset and duration of action.

The onset and duration of action of the insulin preparations is controlled by the size and composition of the crystals in the particular insulin preparation.

> Rapid onset and short duration
>   crystalline zinc insulin (regular)
>   prompt insulin (SEMILENTE)
> Intermediate onset and duration
>   isophane insulin (NPH)
>   insulin zinc (LENTE, mixture of semilente and ultralente)
> Prolonged duration
>   protamine zinc insulin
>   extended insulin zinc (ULTRALENTE)

Basically, insulin is crystallized as a zinc salt. That's where the zinc comes from. The protamine is a positively charged peptide mixture that delays the absorption of the insulin (less soluble complex). In other words, reducing the solubility decreases the absorption and increases the duration of action. Just as an aside, NPH stands for neutral protamine Hagedorn.

ORAL HYPOGLYCEMIC AGENTS

The oral hypoglycemic agents are so named because they lower blood sugar (hypoglycemic) and can be administered orally (as opposed to insulin). That makes the route of administration easy to remember. They are all sulfonylureas, a name that is based on their chemical structure.

> The oral hypoglycemic agents act by stimulating the release of insulin from the β cells in the pancreas.

These agents stimulate insulin release, reduce serum glucagon levels, and increase the binding of insulin to target tissues.

In some books, these drugs are sometimes divided into two groups: first generation and second generation. I should not have to point out that the second generation drugs are newer. The drugs vary in their duration of action and side effects. For now, name recognition is the most important thing for you to learn. Later, if you have time and energy add the "generation" of the drugs. If you are interested, the second generation drugs all start with *g-*.

acetohexamide	GLIPIZIDE
CHLORPROPAMIDE	tolbutamide
gliclazide	tolazamide
GLIBURIDE (glyburide)	

The most common adverse effect of the oral hypoglycemic agents is hypoglycemia.

Hope you can remember that without too much problem.

MISCELLANEOUS DRUGS

·

P A R T   N I N E

MISCELLANEOUS DRUGS

HISTAMINES AND ANTIHISTAMINES

·

Organization of Class

H$_1$ Receptor Antagonists

· · · · · · · · · · · ·

ORGANIZATION OF CLASS

Histamine is an endogenous substance that is widely distributed throughout the body. The physiologic role of histamine is not well understood, but its effects range from itching to anaphylaxis and death. The two principal sites of storage for histamine are the mast cells in tissue and the basophils in blood.

The action of histamine is mediated through at least two receptors: H$_1$ and H$_2$.

H$_3$ receptors have been reported in the brain, but for our purposes there are two classes of histamine receptors.

Intestinal and bronchial smooth muscle contain mostly H_1 receptors. Gastric secretion is mediated by H_2 receptors.

As you can see, the action of histamine depends on the receptors with which it interacts. Histamine itself, or agonists of the histamine receptors, have only minor uses in clinical medicine.

Pharmacological intervention in the action of histamine is currently in the form of receptor antagonists for both the H_1 and H_2 receptors.

Since we will consider drugs that act on the GI tract in a separate chapter, we will not consider the H_2 receptor antagonists any further here.

H_1 RECEPTOR ANTAGONISTS

DIPHENHYDRAMINE	dexbrompheniramine
dimenhydrinate	cyclazine
carbinoxamine	hydroxyzine
tripelennamine	meclizine
pyrilamine	promethazine
chlorpheniramine	cyproheptadine
brompheniramine	TERFENADINE
dexchlorpheniramine	astemizole
clemastine	loratadine

As always, compare the above list with the one in your book or class handouts and make any adjustments. Since many of these agents are available over-the-counter they are more recognizable by their trade names. Next time you are in a drug store spend a few minutes reading the labels on the cold and allergy medicines and see how many of the drug names you recognize.

This group of drugs acts by competitively inhibiting the H_1 receptor.

> The H$_1$ antagonists (antihistamines) are used to treat allergic rhinitis, motion sickness, and sometimes for sleep production.

Note first that this class of drugs is commonly referred to as antihistamines. This is in spite of the fact that there is a whole group of H$_2$ antagonists that could also be called antihistamines, but aren't.

The most common use of antihistamines is in the treatment of runny nose due to seasonal allergies. Most of the antihistamines are lipid-soluble enough to cross the blood–brain barrier. In the CNS they interact with histamine receptors and cause sedation. This effect is sometimes used therapeutically. A number of these drugs are used to treat motion sickness (diphenhydramine, dimenhydrinate, cyclizine, and meclizine). This action may be due to a central antihistamine effect or may be due to a central anticholinergic action. The various agents in this class vary in terms of their anticholinergic potency, the degree of sedation that they induce, and in their duration of action.

> The "nonsedating" antihistamines (TERFENADINE, astemizole, and loratadine) are less lipid-soluble and therefore do not cross the BBB as well. They have less CNS side effects (less sedation).

Be absolutely sure that you know the names of these "nonsedating" antihistamines. Keep in mind that newer ones will probably reach the market in the next few years.

RESPIRATORY DRUGS

·

Organization of Class

β Agonists

Methylxanthines

Cholinergic Antagonists

Cromolyn

·   ·   ·   ·   ·   ·   ·   ·   ·   ·   ·   ·

ORGANIZATION OF CLASS

Bronchoconstriction, inflammation, and loss of lung elasticity are the most common processes that result in respiratory compromise. Bronchoconstriction can be treated with adrenergic agonists, cholinergic antagonists, and some other compounds. Inflammation is treatable with corticosteroids. Obstruction of the airways can also occur with infection and increased secretions. The infection is treated with antibiotics. Since the antibiotics and steroids have been covered elsewhere, this chapter will focus on the bronchodilators. Most of this will be review from the autonomics.

> Drugs used in the treatment of bronchoconstriction include:
>   β agonists
>   cholinergic antagonists
>   methylxanthines

If you then add cromolyn, which is a prophylactic agent, you are all set.

Most of these drugs are now administered by inhalation. This gets the drug to the site of action and this should limit the systemic effects.

β AGONISTS

> β agonists will cause bronchodilation.

β_2-selective agents are preferred to avoid the cardiac effect of β_1 activation.

There are a number of β agonists that are used in the treatment of asthma and chronic obstructive pulmonary disease (COPD).

> β agonists used as bronchodilators:
>   ALBUTEROL
>   metaproterenol
>   TERBUTALINE
>   isoetharine
>   pirbuterol
>   bitolterol

In an emergency, such as the bronchoconstriction associated with anaphylaxis, epinephrine can be used. The nonselective β agonists, iso-proterenol and metaproterenol also are used.

METHYLXANTHINES

The methylxanthines increase cAMP levels, but the exact mechanism by which they cause bronchodilation is not known.

> Aminophylline and THEOPHYLLINE can be used in the treatment of asthma.

Until recently, theophylline or aminophylline was the treatment of choice for the management of asthma. The primary drugs are now the β_2 agonists. Dyphylline is another methylxanthine that some books list. It is rare that students mistake these drugs for another class of compounds. The *phylline* is a dead giveaway.

CHOLINERGIC ANTAGONISTS

The cholinergic antagonists block the bronchoconstriction caused by activation of the parasympathetic nervous system.

> IPRATROPIUM bromide is the DRUG OF CHOICE for the treatment of COPD in adults.

The cholinergic antagonist ipratropium has found use in the treatment of chronic obstructive pulmonary disease (COPD). Ipratropium is less effective against asthma. It is often used in combination with the β agonists.

CROMOLYN

> CROMOLYN sodium is used prophylactically in the treatment of asthma.

Cromolyn is NOT useful in the treatment of an acute attack. The mechanism of action of cromolyn is not clear. It does block the release of mediators from mast cells, but the relevance of this action has been questioned. There is a new relative of cromolyn, called nedocromil sodium.

DRUGS THAT AFFECT THE GI TRACT

·

Organization of Class

Antiulcer Drugs

Antidiarrheals

Pharmacologic Treatment of Constipation

Inflammatory Bowel Disease

Dissolution of Gallstones

·   ·   ·   ·   ·   ·   ·   ·   ·   ·   ·   ·

ORGANIZATION OF CLASS

The organization of these drugs is based on the organization of the GI tract. There are drugs that will treat ulcers in the stomach and duodenum. Then, move on down to the large intestine and divide the agents into those that enhance motility and those that reduce motility.

ANTIULCER DRUGS

Ulcers in the stomach or duodenum are essentially erosion of the mucosa by acid and pepsin. Recently, attention has been drawn to the role of a bacterial infection being the basis of ulcer disease. Medical therapy of ulcer disease mainly consists of neutralizing stomach contents or reducing gastric acid secretions, along with antimicrobial therapy.

H_2 receptor antagonists prevent histamine-induced acid release. H_2 antagonists include:
  CIMETIDINE
  RANITIDINE
  famotidine
  nizatidine

These drugs are easily recognizable by the *-tidine* ending. Hopefully any new drugs that come out will have the same ending. These drugs are used for the short-term treatment of gastroesophageal reflux and peptic ulcer disease.

Antacids are similar in efficacy in treating peptic ulcer disease. The antacids differ in buffering capacity and cost.

The aluminum salts and calcium carbonate antacids cause constipation. The magnesium salts cause diarrhea. Therefore, they are often mixed.

Antacids can decrease the absorption of other drugs because they alter the stomach and duodenal pH. They can also bind to drugs and block their absorption. This is particularly true for the aluminum salts. Antacids also have systemic effects. Magnesium salts can cause hypermagnesemia and aluminum salts can cause hypophosphatemia.

There are a number of other drugs that have been developed for the treatment of ulcer disease that have interesting mechanisms of action.

SUCRALFATE forms a protective coating on the mucosa.

Sucralfate is only minimally absorbed. Constipation is the main side effect.

OMEPRAZOLE inhibits the H^+/K^+ ATPase enzyme of the parietal cell. This reduces acid secretion.

Metoclopramide increases the rate of gastric emptying.

Metoclopramide has both peripheral and central effects. Centrally, it is a dopamine antagonist and it has produced extrapyramidal side effects. Peripherally, it stimulates release of acetylcholine.

MISOPROSTOL is a prostaglandin analog that increases bicarbonate and mucin release and reduces acid secretion. It is used to treat NSAID-induced ulceration.

ANTIDIARRHEALS

Diarrhea is most often caused by infection, toxins, or drugs. Bacterial or parasitic diarrhea should be treated with the appropriate agent for the infection. Drug-induced diarrhea should be treated by discontinuation of the drug, if possible.

Basically, drugs that produce constipation can be used to treat diarrhea. All are given orally. The most common side effect is constipation (surprise!).

Opiates that are used to treat diarrhea include:
DIPHENOXYLATE
LOPERAMIDE

There are also absorbent powders, such as kaolin, a naturally occurring hydrated aluminum silicate, (KAOPECTATE), that are used in the treatment of diarrhea. Bismuth subsalicylate (PEPTO-BISMOL) may coat irritated mucosal surfaces.

PHARMACOLOGIC TREATMENT OF CONSTIPATION

Drugs used to treat constipation can be divided into two groups: the bulk-forming agents and the stimulants and cathartics. These drugs also are taken orally. Some can be administered by insertion into the rectum.

The bulk-forming agents contain plant matter that absorbs water and softens the stool. These include:
   psyllium
   methylcellulose
   calcium polycarbophil

The stimulants increase water and electrolytes in the feces and increase motility. These include:
   bisacodyl
   phenolphthalein
   danthron
   senna

You probably recognize these more by their trade names of METAMUCIL (psyllium), DULCOLAX (bisacodyl), and EX-LAX (phenolphthalein). It helps to remember which are bulk-formers and which are stimulants.

There are a couple of others that you may get asked about. Saline salts of magnesium and sodium (MILK OF MAGNESIA) draw water into the colon. Docusate (COLACE) improves penetration of water and fat into feces.

INFLAMMATORY BOWEL DISEASE

The primary mode of therapy for ulcerative colitis and Crohn's disease utilizes steroids and sulfasalazine.

5-aminosalicylate (5-ASA) is the active metabolite of SULFASALA-ZINE.

Sulfasalazine is metabolized in the colon, by resident bacteria, into 5-ASA and sulfapyridine. The sulfapyridine is absorbed, while the 5-ASA remains in the colon.

DISSOLUTION OF GALLSTONES

Pharmacological dissolution of gallstones is only effective if the stones are made of cholesterol.

Chenodeoxycholic acid and ursodeoxycholic acid, given orally, will dissolve cholesterol stones.

· C H A P T E R · 4 3 ·

NON-NARCOTIC ANALGESICS AND ANTI-INFLAMMATORY DRUGS

·

Organization of Class

NSAIDs

Salicylates, Including Aspirin

Acetaminophen

Gold Preparations

Antigout Agents

· · · · · · · · · · · ·

ORGANIZATION OF CLASS

Some books will put these drugs after the opiate analgesics and other books will put the anti-arthritis drugs together. Basically, we will consider here some salient features of the non-narcotic analgesics and some of the anti-inflammatory agents. The largest group of drugs here is the non-steroidal anti-inflammatory drugs (NSAIDs). This group includes aspirin and the salicylates. However, the salicylates and aspirin have some important special features, so I have separated them to emphasize these features.

NSAIDs

phenylbutazone	NAPROXEN
piroxicam	tolmetin
meclofenamate	diclofenac
INDOMETHACIN	ketoprofen
sulindac	flurbiprofen
IBUPROFEN	etodolac
suprofen	KETOROLAC
fenoprofen	nabumetone
oxaprozin	

Compare this list with the one in your book or class handouts. There seems to be no rhyme or reason for the names.

All the NSAIDs (including aspirin) are thought to exert their clinical effects by inhibiting prostaglandin synthesis.

This is subject to change with further research. The primary site of action is the cyclooxygenase enzyme that catalyzes the conversion of arachidonic acid to prostaglandin and endoperoxide (Fig. 43-1). Prostaglandins modulate components of inflammation, control of body temperature, pain transmission, platelet aggregation, and other effects. They are not stored by cells, but are synthesized and released on demand. Their half-life is not more than minutes. Therefore, if you control the enzyme that makes prostaglandins, then you control the prostaglandins themselves.

The NSAIDs (including aspirin) produce analgesic, antipyretic, anti-inflammatory, and antithrombotic effects.

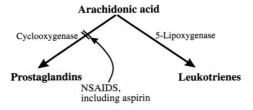

Figure 43-1
Remember that arachidonic acid is converted to both prostaglandins and leukotrienes. The NSAIDs inhibit the enzyme cyclooxygenase and, therefore, the formation of prostaglandins.

The NSAIDs (including aspirin) are used in the treatment of moderate pain, fever, tendinitis, sunburn, rheumatoid arthritis, and osteoarthritis, just to name a few.

> The most common adverse effects of the NSAIDs (including aspirin) are GI injury and renal injury.

GI injury consists of gastritis and ulcers. Misoprostol, a synthetic prostaglandin analog, is used for the prevention of NSAID-induced ulcers. NSAIDs can cause oliguria, fluid retention, decreased sodium excretion, and renal failure. NSAIDs can also prolong bleeding time.

The agents differ with respect to their CNS side effects, duration of action, degree of platelet antagonism (bleeding), and GI toxicity.

> KETOROLAC is a newer NSAID that can be administered intramuscularly or intravenously.

This one may not be in your book yet, but you will see it used in the clinics.

SALICYLATES, INCLUDING ASPIRIN

> The active agent is salicylic acid.

All of these drugs are metabolized to salicylic acid (Fig. 43-2).

Aspirin will bring down a fever, reduce minor pain, reduce inflammation, and prevent blood clots. The antipyretic and analgesic actions are mediated by an action in the CNS. Aspirin has been shown to prevent heart attacks, probably due to its anti-clotting action via inhibition of the production of thromboxane A.

> ASPIRIN, sodium salicylate, and diflunisal are the most commonly used drugs in this group.

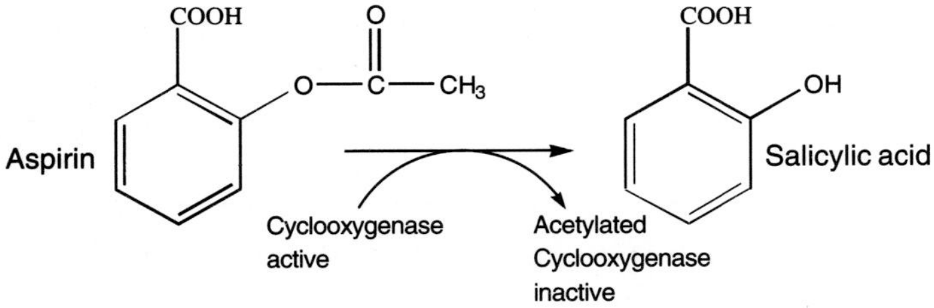

Figure 43-2
Aspirin is metabolized to salicylic acid by the removal of the acetate group. If the acetate is taken by the cyclooxygenase enzyme, then the enzyme is inactivated. In this way aspirin causes an irreversible inhibition of cyclooxygenase.

Use of aspirin has been associated with Reye's syndrome in young children.

Reye's syndrome is characterized by CNS damage, liver injury and hypoglycemia. Its cause is unknown.

Overdose of aspirin is called *salicylism.* Symptoms include ringing in the ears (tinnitus), dizziness, headache, fever, and mental status changes.

Notice that overdose can cause the very symptoms that the patient set out to treat (headache, fever).

The pH changes after ingestion of large amounts of aspirin are complex, but important to understand.
1. Stimulation of the medullary respiratory center causes an increase in ventilation. This leads to RESPIRATORY ALKALOSIS (↑ pH and ↓ pCO_2).
2. There is uncoupling of oxidative phosphorylation. This leads to an increase in plasma CO_2, which further stimulates the respiratory center.

> Aspirin has zero-order kinetics.

Remember zero-order kinetics? Aspirin and salicylic acid are metabolized by glucuronidation—an enzymatic reaction that can be saturated. Therefore, elimination can become zero order (saturation kinetics). This is reflected in the plasma half-life, which increases with increases in dose.

ACETAMINOPHEN

> ACETAMINOPHEN and phenacetin have analgesic and antipyretic actions, but do NOT have anti-inflammatory or antithrombotic activity.

Acetaminophen only weakly inhibits prostaglandin synthesis and has no effect on platelet aggregation.

> ACETAMINOPHEN can cause FATAL liver damage.

In overdose, the major concern is liver damage. This is apparently mediated by the binding of a toxic metabolite to the liver itself (Fig. 43-3). Toxicity can be prevented by intravenous administration of sulfhydryl donors such as N-acetylcysteine, if treatment is initiated quickly.

GOLD PREPARATIONS

> Some gold preparations are used in the treatment of rheumatoid arthritis.

The mechanism of action of these compounds is not known. The most important thing here is to recognize the names.

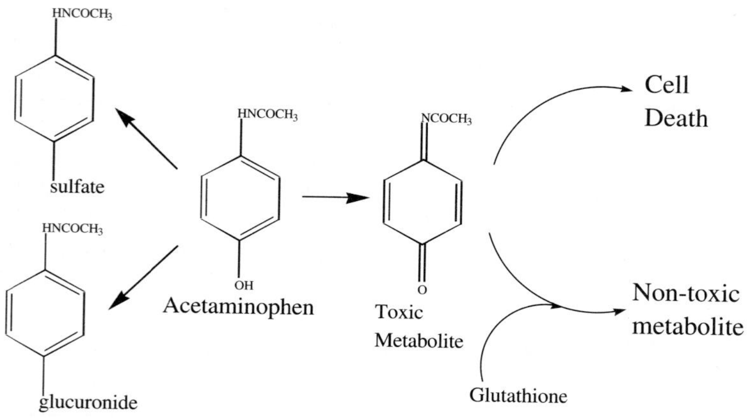

Figure 43-3
Acetaminophen can be metabolized in three directions (arrows). One direction gives a metabolite that is toxic to liver cells. However, glutathione can bind to the toxic metabolite and make it nontoxic. There are only limited quantities of glutathione available. Therefore, high doses of acetaminophen can be toxic.

Auranofin is an orally effective gold preparation.

The other commonly used gold preparations are aurothioglucose and gold sodium thiomalate. If you remember that Au stands for gold on the periodic table (general chemistry, remember?), then you should not have a problem with name recognition.

ANTIGOUT AGENTS

Just a few facts here that you should be sure that you know. Remember that gout is a buildup of uric acid in tissues. Inflammation is due to migration of leukocytes to the joint in an attempt to clean away the uric acid crystals. Pharmacological treatment attempts to increase renal excretion of uric acid by decreasing tubular reabsorption or to decrease synthesis of uric acid (Fig. 43-4).

ALLOPURINOL inhibits xanthine oxidase.

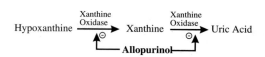

Figure 43-4
Uric acid is formed from hypox-
anthine and xanthine by the enzyme xanthine oxidase. Allopurinol inhibits xanthine oxidase.

Probenecid and sulfinpyrazone inhibit renal reabsorption of uric acid.

Colchicine can be used in acute attacks of gouty arthritis. It reduces
inflammation.

· C H A P T E R · 4 4 ·

IMMUNOSUPPRESSIVES

·

Organization of Class

Cyclosporine

Cytotoxic Drugs

· · · · · · · · · · · ·

ORGANIZATION OF CLASS

Immunopharmacology is the study of the use of drugs to modulate the immune response. The principal application of this field to clinical medicine is with drugs that suppress the immune response. These drugs are used in the treatment of autoimmune diseases and in organ transplantation. Myasthenia gravis and rheumatoid arthritis are examples of autoimmune disorders in which immunosuppressive therapy has been used.

CYCLOSPORINE

CYCLOSPORINE inhibits antibody and cell-mediated immune responses and is the DRUG OF CHOICE for prevention of transplant rejection.

Cyclosporine specifically affects T cells, with little or no effect on B-cell activity. Nephrotoxicity is the major side effect.

FK506 is a newer drug that is similar to cyclosporine.

CYTOTOXIC DRUGS

There are drugs capable of killing immunologically competent cells. These preferentially kill dividing cells, so have the same problems that we discussed for the anticancer drugs.

Azathioprine and cyclophosphamide have been used for immunosuppression.

· C H A P T E R · 4 5 ·

VITAMINS

·

Organization of Class

Fat-Soluble Vitamins

Water-Soluble Vitamins

·   ·   ·   ·   ·   ·   ·   ·   ·   ·   ·   ·

ORGANIZATION OF CLASS

This chapter is included as a reminder of the importance of the vitamins. This material should have been covered in your biochemistry and physiology courses.

Vitamins are a group of chemical substances that are essential for the regulation of normal metabolism, growth, and function of the body.

FAT-SOLUBLE VITAMINS	WATER SOLUBLE VITAMINS
Vitamin A Vitamin D Vitamin E Vitamin K	Vitamin B (including thiamin, riboflavin, niacin, pyridoxine, cyanocobalamin, folic acid and pantothenic acid) Vitamin C

In general, the fat-soluble vitamins are metabolized slowly and stored in the liver. The water-soluble vitamins are metabolized more rapidly and are excreted in the urine.

FAT-SOLUBLE VITAMINS

Vitamin A is used to produce rhodopsin (a visual pigment).

This vitamin is essential for the proper maintenance of epithelial cells.

Vitamin D is a group of compounds involved in calcium homeostasis.

The major source of vitamin D in humans is sunlight irradiation of the skin. Milk is also fortified with vitamin D.

Vitamin E is an antioxidant.

Vitamin K promotes the synthesis of proteins that are involved in coagulation.

WATER-SOLUBLE VITAMINS

Vitamin B is a whole group of substances that tend to occur together in food. Most of the substances are involved in metabolism.

The B vitamins include thiamine, riboflavin, nicotinic acid, pyridoxine, cyanocobalamin, biotin, and folic acid.

Vitamin C acts in the formation and maintenance of collagen.

· I N D E X ·

ABBOKINASE (urokinase), 104
abciximab, 104, 108
ACCUPRIL (quinapril), 76, 97
ACE, 76
ACE inhibitors, 97
acebutolol, 69, 101
acetaminophen, 279
acetohexamide, 258
acetophenazine, 138
acetylcholine, 39, 41
acetylcholinesterase, 41
ACHROMYCIN (tetracycline), 184
ACTH, 239
actinomycin, 222
active transport, 16
acyclovir, 212
ADENOCARD (adenosine), 91
adenosine, 91
adrenal medulla, 41
adrenaline, 41
ADRIAMYCIN (doxorubicin), 222
ADRUCIL (fluorouracil), 223
ADVIL (ibuprofen), 276
afterload, 73, 79
agonist, 9
AIDS, 212
akathisia, 139
AKINETON (biperiden), 121
albuterol, 62, 266
ALDACTONE (spironolactone), 95
ALDOMET (methyldopa), 66, 102
aldosterone, 239
ALEVE (naproxen), 276
alfentanil, 150
ALKERAN (melphalan), 222
alkylating agents, 228
allergy, penicillin, 177

allopurinol, 280
alprazolam, 125, 130
ALTACE (ramipril), 76, 97
aluminum, 270
ALUPENT (metaproterenol), 62, 266
amantadine, 212
ambenonium, 50
amebiasis, 217
AMICAR (aminocaproic acid), 105
AMIDATE (etomidate), 156
amikacin, 182
AMIKIN (amikacin), 182
amiloride, 95
aminocaproic acid, 105, 110
aminoglutethimide, 241
aminoglycosides, 182
aminophylline, 267
aminosalicylic acid, 195
amiodarone, 89
amitriptyline, 132
amlodipine, 80
amobarbital, 125
amoxicillin, 176
AMOXIL (amoxicillin), 176
amphetamine, 63
amphotericin B, 202
ampicillin, 176
amrinone, 75
amyl nitrate, 80
AMYTAL (amobarbital), 125
anabolic, 40
ANCEF (cephazolin), 178
ANCOBON (flucytosine), 202
androgens, 248
ANECTINE (succinylcholine), 56
angina, 79
angiotensin, 76

angiotensin converting enzyme, 76
anisindion, 104
anistreplase, 104, 110
ANSAID (flurbiprofen), 276
antacids, 270
antagonist, 13
anthracyclines, 230
anticoagulant, 105
ANTILIRIUM (physostigmine), 50
antimony, 217
antipsychotics, 137
ANTIVERT (meclizine), 262
ANTURANE (sulfinpyrazone), 104,
    281
ara-A, 212
arachidonic acid, 276
ARALEN (chloroquine), 218
ARDUAN (pipecuronium), 57
arecoline, 49
ARFONAD (trimethaphan), 55
ARISTOCORT (triamcinolone), 238
arrhythmia, 85
ARSOBAL (melarsoprol), 216
ARTANE (trihexylphenidyl), 121
ARTANE (trihexylphenidyl), 54
asparaginase, 223, 226
aspirin, 104, 108, 277
astemizole, 262
asthma, 68, 267
ATABRINE (quinacrine), 216
ATARAX (hydroxyzine), 262
atenolol, 69, 80, 83, 101
ATIVAN (lorazepam), 125
atracurium, 57
ATROMID-S (clofibrate), 114
atropine, 52, 53, 92
ATROVENT (ipratropium), 54, 267
auranofin, 280
AUREOMYCIN (chlotetracycline),
    184
aurothioglucose, 280
autonomic nervous system, 37
AXID (nizatidine), 270
AZACTAM (aztreonam), 179
azathioprine, 284
azithromycin, 185

AZLIN (azlocillin), 176
azlocillin, 176
azole antifungals, 203
AZT, 212
aztreonam, 174, 179
AZULFIDINE (sulfasalazine), 190,
    272

bacitracin, 180
bactericidal, 169
bacteriostatic, 169
BACTRIM (co-trimoxazole), 190
barbiturates, 124
    withdrawal, 127
BCNU (carmustine), 222
benazepril, 76, 97
BENEMID (probenecid), 281
BENTYL (dicyclomine), 54
benzathine pen G, 176
benzocaine, 162
benzodiazepines, 124
    dependence, 129
    half-life, 128
    metabolism, 127
benztropine, 121
benztropine, 54
bepridil, 80
betamethasone, 238
BETAPACE (sotalol), 89
betaxolol, 69, 101
bethanechol, 49
BIAXIN (clarithromycin), 185
BILTRICIDE (praziquantel), 208
bioavailability, 18
biperiden, 121
bisacodyl, 272
bismuth subsalicylate, 272
bisoprolol, 69
bitolterol, 266
BLENOXANE (bleomycin), 222
bleomycin, 222, 226, 231
BONINE (meclizine), 262
botulinum toxin, 57
BRETHAIRE (terbutaline), 62, 266
bretylium, 89

BREVIBLOC (esmolol), 101
BREVITAL (methohexital), 125
bromocriptine, 121
brompheniramine, 262
BRONKSOL (isoetharine), 266
bumetanide, 95
BUMEX bumetanide), 95
bupivacaine, 162
buprenorphine, 150
BUSPAR (busprione), 125
buspirone, 125, 130
busulfan, 222
BUTAZOLID (phenylbutazone), 276
butoconazole, 202
butorphanol, 150

CALAN (verapamil), 80
calcium channel blockers, 82, 90, 99
calcium polycarbophil, 272
CAPASTAT (capreomycin), 195
CAPOTEN (captopril), 76, 97
capreomycin, 195
captopril, 76, 97
CARAFATE (sucralfate), 270
carbachol, 49
carbamazepine, 144
carbenicillin, 176
carbidopa, 121
carbinoxamine, 262
CARBOCAINE (mepivacaine), 162
carboplatin, 223, 233
CARDENE (nicardipine), 80
cardiotoxicity, 227
CARDIZEM (diltiazem), 80
CARDURA (doxazosin), 67, 100
carmustine, 222, 229
carteolol, 69, 101
CARTROL (carteolol), 69, 101
catabolic, 40
CATAPRES (clonidine), 61, 66, 102
catecholamine, 42
CCNU (lomustine), 222
CECLOR (cefaclor), 178
cefaclor, 178
cefamandole, 178

cefazolin, 178
cefotaxime, 178
cefoxitin, 178
ceftazidine, 178
ceftriaxone, 178
cell cycle, 224
cephalexin, 178
cephalosporins, 174, 178
CERUBIDINE (daunarubicin), 222
cestodes, 208
Chagas' disease, 217
chenodeoxycholic acid, 273
chlamydia, 184, 186
chloral hydrate, 125
chlorambucil, 222, 228
chloramphenicol, 182, 186
chlordiazepoxide, 125, 129
CHLOROMYCETIN
  (chloramphenicol), 186
chloroquine, 218
chlorothalidone, 95
chlorothiazide, 95
chlorpheniramine, 262
chlorprocaine, 162
chlorpromazine, 138, 226, 258
CHLORTRIMETON
  (chlorpheniramine), 262
chlotetracycline, 184
cholera, 184
cholesterol, 113, 273
cholesterol synthesis, 114
cholestyramine, 114
cholinesterases, 48
cholinomimetics, 47
cilastatin, 179
cimetidine, 270
cinchonism, 220
CIPRO (ciprofloxacin), 191
ciprofloxacin, 191
cisplatin, 223, 233
cladribine, 223
CLAFORAN (cefotaxime), 178
CLARATIN (loratidine), 262
clarithromycin, 185
clavulinic acid, 175
clearance, 19, 24

clemastine, 262
CLEOCIN (clindamycin), 187
clindamycin, 182, 187
CLINORIL (sulindac), 276
clofibrate, 114
CLOMID (clomiphene), 244
clomiphene, 244
clonazepam, 125, 147
clonidine, 61, 66, 102
clorazepate, 125
clotrimazole, 202
cloxacillin, 176
clozapine, 138, 140
CLOZARIL (clozapine), 138, 140
cocaine, 162
codeine, 150, 152
COGENTIN (benztropine), 121
COLASE (docusate), 272
colchicine, 281
COLESTID (colestipol), 114
colestipol, 114
COMPAZINE (prochlorperazine), 138
competitive antagonist, 13
COMT, 41
CORDARONE (amiodarone), 89
CORGARD (nadolol), 69
cortisol, 238
COSMEGEN (dactinomycin), 222
COUMADIN (warfarin), 104
craniosacral, 40
Crohn's, 272
cromolyn, 267
cross-dependence, 124
cross-tolerance, 124
CRYSTODIGIN (digitoxin), 74
CUTOXAN (cyclophosphamide), 222,
    284
cyanocobalamin, 105
cyclazine, 262
cyclooxygenase, 108, 278
cyclopentolate, 54
cyclophosphamide, 222, 228, 284
cycloserine, 195
cyclosporine, 283
CYKLOKAPRON (tranexamic acid),
    110

cyproheptadine, 262
cyproterone, 244
CYTADREN (aminoglutethimide),
    241
cytarabine, 223, 230
CYTOSAR-U (cytarabine), 223
CYTOTEC (misoprostol), 271
CYTOVENE (ganciclovir), 212

dacarbazine, 222
dactinomycin, 222
DALMANE (flurazepam), 125
danazol, 244
DANOCRINE (danazol), 244
danthron, 272
dantrolene, 57
dapsone, 198
DARAPRIM (pyrimethamine), 218
DARVON (propoxyphene), 150
daunarubicin, 222
daunomycin, 222
daunorubicin, 230
DAYPRO (oxaprozin), 276
DDC, 212
DDI, 212
DECADRON (dexamethasone), 238
DECLOMYCIN (demeclocycline), 184
dehydroemetine, 216
DELTASONE (predisone), 238
demecarium, 50
demeclocycline, 184
DEMEROL (meperidine), 150
DENDRID (idoxuridine), 212
DEPAKENE (valproic acid), 144
dependence, 124
DEPO-MEDROL
    (methylprednisolone), 238
deprenyl, 121
desipramine, 132
dexamethasone, 238
dexbrompheniramine, 262
DEXEDRINE (amphetamine), 63
diabetes insipidus, 255
    mellitus, 255
diabetics, 68

DIABINASE (chlorpropamide), 258
diazepam, 125, 129, 160
diazoxide, 99
DIBENZYLINE (phenoxybenzamine), 67
diclofenac, 276
dicloxacillin, 176
dicumarol, 104
dicyclomine, 54
didanosine, 212
diethylcarbamazine, 209
diethylstilbestrol, 244
DIFLUCAN (fluconazole), 202
diflunisal, 278
digitalis, 74
digitoxin, 74
digoxin, 74, 91
dihydrocodeine, 150
diisopropyl flurophosphate, 50
DILANTIN (phenytoin), 87, 144
DILAUDID (hydromorphone), 150
diltiazem, 80
dimenhydrinate, 262
DIMETABS (dimenhydrinate), 262
diphenhydramine, 262
diphenoxylate, 271
diphtheria, 186
DIPRIVAN (propofol), 156
dipyridamole, 104, 108
disopyramide, 87
DISTOCIDE (praziquantel), 208
DITROPAN (oxybutynin), 54
diuretics, 95
DIURIL (chlorothiazide), 95
dobutamine, 62, 77
DOBUTREX (dobutamine), 62, 77
DOLOBID (diflunisal), 278
DOLOPHINE (methadone), 150
DOMALIN (quazepam), 125
dopamine, 62, 77
  in Parkinson's, 119
doxacurium, 57
doxazosin, 67, 100
doxepine, 132
doxorubicin, 222, 230
doxycycline, 184

DRAMAMINE (dimenhydrinate), 262
DTIC-DOME (dacarbazine), 222
DULCOLAX (bisacodyl), 272
DURANEST (etidocaine), 162
DYMELOR (acetohexamide), 258
DYNACIRC (isradipine), 80
dystonia, 139

echothiophate, 50
econazole, 202
EDECRIN (ethacrynic acid), 95
edrophonium, 50, 51
efficacy, 10
eflornithine, 216
EFUDEX (fluorouracil), 223
ELAVIL (amitriptyline), 132
ELDEPRYL (selegiline or deprenyl), 121
elimination rate constant, 23
ELSPAR (asparaginase), 223
EMCYT (estramustine), 223
emetine, 216
EMINASE (anistreplase), 104
enalapril, 76, 97
encainide, 87
endometriosis, 248
enflurane, 156
enoxacin, 191
ephedrine, 62
epilepsy, 143
epinephrine, 41, 60, 63, 92
epoetin alpha, 105, 111
EPOGEN (epoetin alpha), 105
ergosterol, 203
ERYCETTE (erythromycin), 185
erythromycin, 182, 185
erythropoietin, 105, 111
ESKALITH (lithium), 135
ESMILIL (quanethidine), 101
esmolol, 69, 101
estradiol, 244
estramustine, 223
estriol, 244
estrogen, 232

estrone, 244
ethacrynic acid, 95
ethambutol, 195
ethinyl estradiol, 244
ethionamide, 195
ETHMOZINE (moricizine), 91
ethosuximide, 144
ETHRANE (enflurane), 156
etidocaine, 162
etodolac, 276
etomidate, 156, 160
etoposide, 222, 232
EULEXIN (flutamide), 223, 244
EUTHROID (liotrix), 252
EXLAX (phenolphthalein), 272
extrapyramidal effects, 139

famciclovir, 212
famotidine, 270
FAMVIR (famciclovir), 212
FELDENE (piroxicam), 276
felodipine, 80
FEMSTAT (butoconazole), 202
fenoprofen, 276
fentanyl, 150, 153
filaria, 209
filgrastim, 223, 234
finasteride, 244, 248
first pass effect, 15
first-order, 23
FLAGYL (metronidazole), 216
flecainide, 87
FLOROPRYL (isopflurophate), 50
flosequin, 76
FLOXIN (ofloxacin), 191
fluconazole, 202
flucytosine, 202, 204
FLUDARA (fludarabine), 223
fludarabine, 223
fludrocortisone, 238
flukes, 208
FLUMADINE (rimantadine), 212
flumazenil, 129
FLUORINEF (fludrocortisone), 238
fluorouracil, 223, 230
FLUOTHANE (halothane), 156

fluoxetine, 132
fluoxymesterone, 244
fluphenazine, 138
flurazepam, 125, 130
flurbiprofen, 276
flutamide, 223, 232, 244
fluvastatin, 114
folate antagonists, 189
folic acid, 105, 110
FORANE (isoflurane), 156
formaldehyde, 193
FORTAZ (ceftazidine), 178
fosinopril, 76, 97
FULVIN (griseofulvin), 202
FUNGIZONE (amphotericin), 202
FURADANTIN (nitrofurantoin), 191
furosemide, 95

GABA, 125
gallamine, 57
ganciclovir, 212
GANTANEL (sulfamethoxazole), 190
GANTRISIN (sulfisoxazole), 190
GARAMYCIN (gentamicin), 182
gemfibrozil, 114
gentamicin, 182
GEOPEN (carbenicillin), 176
giardia, 217
glaucoma, 52
gliburide, 258
gliclazide, 258
glipizide, 258
glomerular filtration, 34
glucocorticoids, 240
GLUCOTROL (glipizide), 258
glyburide, 258
glycopyrrolate, 54
glycosides, cardiac, 74
gold sodium thiomalate, 280
GRIFULVIN (griseofulvin), 202
griseofulvin, 202
griseofulvin, 205
growth factors, 234
guanabenz, 66, 102
guanadrel, 101

guanethidine, 101
guanfacine, 66

HALCION (triazolam), 125
HALDOL (haloperidol), 138
half-life, 23
haloperidol, 138
HALOTESTIN (fluoxymesterone), 244
halothane, 156, 159
helminths, 207
heparin, 104, 106
heroin, 150, 152
HERPLEX (idoxuridine), 212
hexamethonium, 55
HISMANAL (astemizole), 262
histamine, 261
HIV, 212
HIVID (zalcitabine), 212
HMG CoA reductase, 114
hookworm, 209
HUMORSOL (demecarium), 50
HUMULIN (insulin), 257
hydralazine, 99
HYDREA (hydroxyurea), 223
hydrochlorothiazide, 95
hydrocodone, 150
hydrocortisone, 238
hydromorphone, 150
hydroxychloroquine, 218
hydroxyprogesterone, 244
hydroxyurea, 223, 233
hydroxyzine, 262
HYLOREL (quanadrel), 101
hypercalcemia, 231
HYTRIN (terazosin), 67, 100

ibuprofen, 276
IDAMYCIN (idarubicin), 222
idarubicin, 222
idoxuridine, 212
IFEX (ifosfamide), 222
ifosfamide, 222
ILOTYCIN (erythromycin), 185
imipenem, 174, 179

imipramine, 132
IMODIUM (loperamide), 271
IMURAN (azathioprine), 284
indapamide, 95
indecainide, 87
INDERAL (propranolol), 69, 80, 89, 101
INDOCIN (indomethacin), 276
indomethacin, 276
influenza, 213
infusion rate, 27
INH (isoniazid), 195
inhibitory concentration, 172
INOCOR (amrinone), 75
insulin, 256
interferon, 223
intrinsic factor, 111
INVERSINE (mecamylamine), 55
iodoquinol, 216
ipratropium, 54, 267
iron, 105, 110
ISMELIN (quanethidine), 101
isocarboxazid, 132, 134
isoetharine, 266
isoflurane, 156, 159
isoflurophate, 50
isoniazid, 195
isoproterenol, 62, 64, 92
ISOPTIN (verapamil), 80
isosorbide dinitrate, 80
isosorbide mononitrate, 80
isradipine, 80
ISUPREL (isoproterenol), 62
itraconazole, 202
ivermectin, 209

K$^+$-sparing diuretics, 97
KABIKINASE (streptokinase), 104
kanamycin, 182, 195
KANTREX (kanamycin), 182
KEFLEX (cephalexin), 178
KERLONE (betaxolol), 69
KETALAR (ketamine), 156
ketamine, 156, 160
ketoconazole, 202, 241

ketoprofen, 276
ketorolac, 276, 277
KLONOPIN (clonazepam), 125, 147

labetalol, 69, 100
LAMPIT (nifurtimox), 216
LANOXIN (digoxin), 74, 91
LARIAM (mefloquine), 218
LASIX (furosemide), 95
Legionnaire's, 186
leishmaniasis, 217
LENTE (insulin), 257
leprosy, 195, 198
leucovorin, 229
LEUKERAN (chlorambucil), 222
leuprolide, 223, 233
LEUSTATIN (cladribine), 223
LEVATOL (penbutolol), 69, 101
LEVO-DROMORAN (levorphanol), 150
levobunolol, 69
levodopa, 120
LEVOPHED (norepinephrine), 60
levorphanol, 150
LEVOTHYROID (thyroxine), 252
levothyroxine, 252
LEVOXINE (thyroxine), 252
LIBRIUM (chlordiazepoxide), 125
lidocaine, 87, 162
lincomycin, 187
lincosamides, 187
liothyronine, 252
liotrix, 252
lipoprotein, 113
lisinopril, 76, 97
lithium, 135
loading dose, 30
LODINE (etodolac), 276
log kill, 224
lomefloxacin, 191
LOMOTIL (diphenoxylate), 271
lomustine, 222, 229
loop diuretics, 96
loperamide, 271
LOPID (gemfibrozil), 114

LOPRESSOR (metoprolol), 69
loratadine, 262
lorazepam, 125, 160
LORELCO (probucol), 114
losartan, 99
LOTENSIN (benazepril), 76, 97
LOTRIMIN (clotrimazole), 202
lovastatin, 114
loxapine, 138
LOZOL (indapamide), 95
LUDIOMIL (maprotiline), 132
LUPRON (leuprolide), 223, 233
Lyme disease, 184
LYSODREN (mitotane), 223

MAC, 158
macrolides, 182, 185
magnesium, 91
major tranquilizers, 137
malaria, 217
malathion, 50
MANDOL (cefamandole), 178
MAO, 42
MAO inhibitors, 134
maprotiline, 132
MARCAINE (bupivacaine), 162
MAREZINE (cyclizine), 262
MARPLAN (isocarboxazid), 132
MATULANE (procarbazine), 223
MAXAIRE (pirbuterol), 266
MAXAQUIN (lomefloxacin), 191
mebendazole, 209
mecamylamine, 55
mechlorethamine, 222, 228
meclizine, 262
meclofenamate, 276
MECLOMEN (meclofenamate), 276
medroxyprogesterone, 244
mefloquine, 218
MEFOXIN (cefoxitin), 178
megaloblastic anemia, 111
megestrol, 244
melarsoprol, 216
MELLARIL (thioridazine), 138
melphalan, 222

meperidine, 150, 152
MEPHYTON (vitamin K), 105
mepivacaine, 162
meprobamate, 125
mercaptopurine, 230
mesoridazine, 138
MESTINON (pyridostigmine), 50
mestranol, 244
metabolism, 33
METAMUCIL (psyllium), 272
METAPREL (metaproterenol), 62
metaprolol, 101
metaproterenol, 62, 266
methacholine, 49
methadone, 150, 153
methenamine, 191
methicillin, 176
methimazole, 253
methohexital, 125, 160
methotrexate, 189, 223, 229
methoxyflurane, 156
methylcellulose, 272
methyldopa, 66, 102
methylphenidate, 63
methylprednisolone, 238
methyltestosterone, 244
metoclopramide, 271
metocurine iodide, 57
metolazone, 95
metoprolol, 69, 80, 83
metronidazole, 216
metyrapone, 241
MEVACOR (lovastatin), 114
MEXATE (methotrexate), 189, 223, 229
mexiletine, 87
MEXITIL (mexiletine), 87
MEZLIN (mazlocillin), 176
mezlocillin, 176
MIC, 172
miconazole, 202
MICRONASE (glyburide), 258
microtubules, 232
midazolam, 160
mifepristone, 244, 247
milrinone, 75

mineralocorticoids, 241
MINIPRESS (prazosin), 67, 100
MINOCIN (minocycline), 184
minocycline, 184
minoxidil, 99
MINTEZOL (thiabendazole), 209
miosis, 45
misoprostol, 271, 277
MITHRACIN (plicamycin), 222
mithramycin, 222, 231
mitomycin, 222
mitotane, 223, 233
mitoxantrone, 223
MIVACRON (mivacurium), 57
MODANE (danthron), 272
MONISTAT (miconazole), 202
monobactam, 179
mononucleosis, 177
MONOPRIL (fosinopril), 76, 97
moricizine, 87, 91
morphine, 150
motion sickness, 263
MOTRIN (ibuprofen), 276
muscarine, 40, 43, 48, 49
MUSTARGEN (mechlorethamine), 222
MUTAMYCIN (mitomycin), 222
muzolimine, 95
MYAMBUTOL (ethambutol), 195
myasthenia gravis, 51
MYCELEX (clotrimazole), 202
mycobacteria, 195
mycoplasma, 184
MYCOSTATIN (nystatin), 202
mydriasis, 45
MYLERAN (busulfan), 222
MYSOLINE (primidone), 144

nabumetone, 276
nadolol, 69, 80, 83, 101
NAFCIL (nafcillin), 176
naftifine, 202
NAFTIN (naftifine), 202
nalbuphine, 150
NALFON (fenoprofen), 276

nalidixic acid, 191
naloxone, 150, 154
naltrexone, 150
NAPROSYN (naproxen), 276
NARCAN (naloxone), 150
narcotic, withdrawal, 152
narcotics, 149
NARDIL (phenelzine), 132
NAVANE (thiothixene), 138
NEBCIN (tobramycin), 182
NEGGRAM (nalidixic acid), 191
nematodes, 209
NEMBUTAL (pentobarbital), 125
neomycin, 182
NEOSPORIN (bacitracin), 180
neostigmine, 50
NEOSYNEPHRINE (phenylephrine),
    61
nephrotoxicity, 183
netilmicin, 182
NETROMYCIN (netilmicin), 182
NEUPOGEN (filgrastim), 223
neuroleptic malignant syndrome,
    141
neuroleptics, 137
neurotoxicity, 183
niacin, 114
nicardipine, 80
NICLOCIDE (niclosamide), 208
niclosamide, 208
nicotine, 50
nicotinic, 43
nifedipine, 80
nifurtimox, 216
nimodipine, 80
NIMOTOP (nimodipine), 80
nitrates, 80
nitrofurantoin, 191
nitrogen mustards, 228
nitroglycerin, 80
nitroprusside, 100
nitrous oxide, 156, 159
nizatidine, 270
NIZORAL (ketoconazole), 202
NOLVADEX (tamoxifen), 223,
    244

noncompetitive antagonist, 14
noradrenaline, 41
NORCURON (vecuronium), 57
norepinephrine, 41, 60, 63
norethindrone, 244
norfloxacin, 191
norgestrol, 244
NORMODYNE (labetalol), 69
NOROXIN (norfloxacin), 191
NORPACE (disopyramide), 87
NORPRAMIN (desipramine), 132
nortriptyline, 132
NORVASC (amlodipine), 80
NOVANTRONE (mitoxantrone), 223
NOVOCAINE (procaine), 162
NPH (insulin), 257
NUBAIN (nalbuphine), 150
NUPRINM (ibuprofen), 276
NUROMAX (doxacurium), 57
nystatin, 202
nystatin, 206

OCUFLOX (ofloxacin), 191
ofloxacin, 191
omeprazole, 271
OMNIPEN (ampicillin), 176
onchoceriasis, 210
ONCOVIN (vincristine), 222
ondansetron, 226
opiates, 149
optic neuritis, 198
oral contraceptives, 247
ORINASE (tolbutamide), 258
ORNIDYL (eflornithine), 216
ORUDIS (ketoprofen), 276
ototoxicity, 183
oxacillin, 176
oxaprozin, 276
oxazepam, 125
oxiconazole, 202
OXISTAT (oxiconzaole), 202
oxybutynin, 54
oxycodone, 150
oxymorphone, 150
oxytetracycline, 184

PABA, 189
paclitaxel, 222
paclitaxel, 232
pancuronium, 57
paramethasone, 238
PARAPLATIN (carboplatin), 223
parasympathetic, 40, 44
parathion, 50
Parkinson's Disease, 119
Parkinsonism, 139
PARLODEL (bromocriptine), 121
PARNATE (tranylcypromine), 132
paroxetine, 132
partial agonist, 10
partial pressure, 156
passive diffusion, 16
PATHOCIL (dicloxacillin), 176
PAVULON (pancuronium), 57
PAXIL (paroxetine), 132
PBZ (tripelennamine), 262
PDE inhibitors, 75
peak, 28
penbutolol, 101
penbutolol, 69
PENETREX (enoxacin), 191
penicillin G, 176
penicillin V, 176
penicillin-binding proteins, 174
penicillins, 174
PENTAM (pentamidine), 216
pentamidine, 216
pentapril, 76, 97
pentazocine, 150, 154
PENTIDS (penicillin G), 176
pentobarbital, 125
PENTOSTAM (sodium
    stibogluconate), 216
pentostatin, 223
PEPCID (famotidine), 270
PEPTO-BISMOL, 272
pergolide, 121
PERIACTIN (cyproheptadine), 262
PERMAX (pergolide), 121
pernicious anemia, 111
perphenazine, 138
pertussis, 186

phenacetin, 279
phenelzine, 132, 134
PHENERGAN (promethazine), 262
phenobarbital, 125, 144, 146
phenolphthalein, 272
phenoxybenzamine, 67
phentolamine, 67
phenylbutazone, 276
phenylephrine, 61
phenylpropanolamine, 62
phenytoin, 87, 144
phenytoin, kinetics, 145
phosphodiesterase, 76
PHOSPHOLINE (echothiophate), 50
photosensitivity, 185
physostigmine, 50
pilocarpine, 49
pinacidil, 99
pindolol, 69, 101
pinworm, 209
pipecuronium, 57
piperacillin, 176
PIPRACEL (piperacillin), 176
pirbuterol, 266
pirenzepine, 54
piroxicam, 276
PLAQUENIL (hydroxychloroquine),
    218
plasmids, 170
plasmodium, 217
PLATINOL (cisplatin), 223
PLENDIL (felodipine), 80
plicamycin, 222, 231
polyene antifungals, 203
POLYSPORIN (bacitracin), 180
PONTOCAINE (tetracaine), 162
postganglionic, 39
potency, 10
pralidoxime, 52
PRAVACHOL (pravastatin), 114
pravastatin, 114
praziquantel, 208
prazosin, 67, 100
prednisolone, 238
prednisone, 238
preganglionic, 39

preload, 73
prilocaine, 162
PRILOSEC (omeprazole), 271
PRIMACOR (milrinone), 75
primaquine, 218
PRIMAXIN (imipenem-cilastatin), 179
primidone, 144, 147
PRINIVIL (lisinopril), 76, 97
PRISCOLINE (tolazoline), 67
probenecid, 176, 281
probucil, 115
probucol, 114
procainamide, 87
procaine, 162
PROCAN (procainamide), 87
procarbazine, 223
PROCARDIA (nifedipine), 80
prochlorperazine, 138
progesterone, 244
prolactin, 139
PROLIXIN (fluphenazine), 138
promethazine, 262
propafenone, 87
propantheline, 54
propofol, 156, 160
propoxyphene, 150
propranolol, 69, 80, 83, 89, 101
propylthiouracil, 253
PROSCAR (finasteride), 244, 248
prostaglandin, 276
PROSTAPHLIN (oxacillin), 176
prostatic hypertrophy, 248
PROSTIGMIN (neostigmine), 50
protamine, 106
protamine sulfate, 105
PROTOPAM (pralidoxime), 52
PROTOSTAT (metronidazole), 216
PROVENTIL (albuterol), 62, 266
PROVOCHOLINE (methacholine), 49
PROZAC (fluoxetine), 132
pseudocholinesterase, 48
psyllium, 272
pulmonary fibrosis, 228
PURINETHOL (mercaptopurine), 223
pyrazinamide, 195
pyridostigmine, 50

pyrilamine, 262
pyrimethamine, 189, 218

quazepam, 125
QUELICIN (succinylcholine), 56
QUESTRAN (cholestyramine), 114
quinacrine, 216
QUINAGLUTE (quindiine), 87
quinapril, 76, 97
quinestrol, 244
quinidine, 87
quinine, 218
quinolones, 191

radioactive iodine, 253
ramipril, 76, 97
ranitidine, 270
REGITINE (phentolamine), 67
REGLAN (metoclopramide), 271
RELAFEN (nabumetone), 276
renin, 76
reserpine, 101
resistance, bacterial, 169
respiratory syncytial virus, 213
RESTORIL (temazepam), 125
RETROVIR (zidovudine), 212
retrovirus, 212
Reye's syndrome, 278
ribavirin, 212
ribosomes, 181
rickettsia, 184
RIDAURA (auranofin), 280
RIFADIN (rifampin), 195
rifampin, 195
RIFATER (pyrazinamide), 195
RIMACTANE (rifampin), 195
rimantadine, 212
RITALINE (methylphenidate), 63
ROBINUL (glycopyrrolate), 54
ROCEPHIN (ceftriaxone), 178
Rocky Mountain Spotted Fever, 184
rocurium, 57
ROGAINE (minoxidil), 99
ROMAZICON (flumazenil), 129

ropivacaine, 162
roundworms, 209
ROXANOL (morphine), 150
RUFEN (ibuprofen), 276
RYTHMOL (propafenone), 87

SALAGEN (pilocarpine), 49
salicylic acid, 277
salicylism, 278
salivary glands, 44
SANDIMMUNE (cyclosporine), 283
saralasin, 98
sargramostim, 223, 234
sarin, 50
scopolamine, 54
secobarbital, 125
SECONAL (secobarbital), 125
SECTRAL (acebutolol), 69, 101
seizures, 143
SELDANE (terfenadine), 262
selegiline, 121
SEMILENTE (insulin), 257
semustine, 222, 229
senna, 272
SENSORCAINE (bupivacaine), 162
SEPTRA (co-trimoxazole), 190
SERAX (oxazepam), 125
SEROMYCIN (cycloserine), 195
sertraline, 132
simvastatin, 114
SINEMET (carbidopa and levodopa),
    121
SINEQUAN (doxepin), 132
SLO-PHYLLIN (theophylline), 267
SOLGANGAL (aurothioglucose), 280
soman, 50
sotalol, 89
spectrum, 169
SPEXTAZOLE (econazole), 202
spirochetes, 184
spironolactone, 95, 241
SPORANOX (itraconazole), 202
SSRIs, 133
STADOL (butorphanol), 150
STAPHCILLIN (methicillin), 176

steady-state, 27
    time to reach, 28
STELAZINE (trifluoperazine), 138
sterol, 203
stibogluconate, 216
STILPHOSTROL (diethylstilbestrol),
    244
STOXIL (idoxuridine), 212
streptokinase, 104, 109
streptomycin, 182, 195
SUBLIMAZE (fentanyl), 150
succinylcholine, 56
sucralfate, 270
sufentanil, 150
sulbactam, 175
sulfacetamide, 190
sulfadiazine, 190
sulfamethoxazole, 190
sulfapyridine, 190
sulfasalazine, 190, 272
Sulfinpyrazone, 104, 108, 281
sulfisoxazole, 190
sulfonamides, 189
sulindac, 276
superinfection, 170
suprofen, 276
suramin, 216
SYMMETREL (amantadine), 212
sympathetic, 40, 44
SYNTHROID (thyroxine), 252

t-PA, 104, 109
TAGAMET (cimetidine), 270
TALWIN (pentazocine), 150
TAMBOCOR (flecainide), 87
tamoxifen, 223, 232, 244
TAPAZOLE (methimazole), 253
tapeworms, 208
tardive dyskinesia, 139
TAVIST (clemastine), 262
TAXOL (paclitaxel), 222
TAZICEF (ceftazidine), 178
tazobactam, 175
TEGOPEN (cloxacillin), 176
TEGRETOL (carbamazepine), 144

teicoplanin, 179
temazepam, 125, 130
TEMPRA (acetaminophen), 279
TENEX (guanfacine), 66
teniposide, 222, 232
TENORMIN (atenolol), 69
TENSILON (edrophonium), 50
TERAZOL (terconazole), 202
terazosin, 67, 100
terbutaline, 62, 266
terconazole, 202
terfenadine, 262
TERRAMYCIN (oxytetracycline), 184
testosterone, 232, 244, 248
tetracaine, 162
tetracycline, 184
tetracyclines, 182
tetracyclines, 184
THEO-DUR (theophylline), 267
theophylline, 267
therapeutic index, 12
therapeutic window, 12
thiabendazole, 209
thiamylal, 160
thiazide diuretics, 96
THIOGUAN (thioguanine), 223
thioguanine, 223, 230
thiopental, 125, 156, 160
thioridazine, 138
thiotepa, 222
thiothixene, 138
thoracolumbar, 40
THORAZINE (chlorpromazine), 138
thyroglobulin, 251
THYROLAR (liotrix), 252
TICAR (ticarcillin), 176
ticarcillin, 176
TICLID (ticlopidine), 104
ticlopidine, 104, 108
timolol, 69, 101
tobramycin, 182
tocainide, 87
TOFRANIL (imipramine), 132
tolazamide, 258
tolazoline, 67
tolbutamide, 258

TOLECTIN (tolmetin), 276
tolerance, 123
TOLINASE (tolazamide), 258
tolmetin, 276
tolnaftate, 202
TONOCARD (tocainide), 87
TORADOL (ketorolac), 276
TORNALATE (bitolterol), 266
TRACRIUM (atracurium), 57
TRANDATE (labetalol), 69
tranexamic acid, 105, 110
transposons, 170
TRANXENE (clorazepate), 125
tranylcypromine, 132, 134
TRECATOR-SC (ethionamide), 195
trematodes, 208
TREXAN (naltrexone), 150
triamcinolone, 238
triamterine, 95
triazolam, 125, 130
trichomoniasis, 216
trifluoperazine, 138
trihexylphenidyl, 54, 121
trimazosin, 67
trimethaphan, 55
trimethoprim, 190
trimoxazole, 190
TRIMPEX (trimethoprim), 190
tripelennamine, 262
tropicamide, 54
trough, 28
trypanosomiasis, 217
tuberculosis, 195
tubocurarine, 57
tubular reabsorption, 34
tubular secretion, 34
tubulin, 231
TYLENOL (acetaminophen), 279
tyramine, 134

ulcer, 269
ulcerative colitis, 272
ULTRALENTE (insulin), 257
URECHOLINE (bethanechol), 49
uric acid, 280

URISED (methenamine), 191
URO-PHOSPHATE (methenamine), 191
urokinase, 104, 109
ursodeoxycholic acid, 273

VALIUM (diazepam), 125
valproic acid, 144, 146
VANCOCIN (vancomycin), 179
vancomycin, 174, 179
VASCOR (bepridil), 80
VASOTEC (enalapril), 76, 97
vecuronium, 57
VEETIDS (penicillin V), 176
VELBAN (vinblastine), 222
VELSAR (vinblastine), 222
VENTOLIN (albuterol), 62, 266
VEPESIOL (etoposide), 222
verapamil, 80
VERMOX (mebendazole), 209
VIBRAMYCIN (doxycycline), 184
vidarabine, 212
VIDEX (didanosine), 212
vinblastine, 222, 231
VINCASAR (vinctristine), 222
vincristine, 222, 231
viomycin, 195
VIRA-A (vidarabine), 212
VIRAZOLE (ribavirin), 212
VISTARIL (hydroxyzine), 262
vitamin K, 105, 107

VOLTAREN (diclofenac), 276
volume of distribution, 21
VUMOR (teniposide), 222

warfarin, 104, 107
whipworm, 209
withdrawal, 124
WYTENSIN (guanabenz), 66

XANAX (alprazolam), 125
XYLOCAINE (lidocaine), 87, 162

YOCON (yohimbine), 67
YODOXIN (iodoquinol), 216

zalcitabine, 212
ZANTAC (ranitidine), 270
ZARONTIN (ethosuximide), 144
ZAROXOLYN (metolazone), 95
zero order, 25
ZESTRIL (lisinopril), 76, 97
zidovudine, 212
ZITHROMAX (azithromycin), 185
ZOCOR (simvastatin)i, 114
ZOLOFT (sertraline), 132
zolpidem, 130
ZOVIRAX (acyclovir), 212
ZYLOPRIM (allopurinol), 280